A NEURODEVELOPMENTAL PERSPECTIVE ON SPECIFIC LEARNING DISABILITIES

A NEURODEVELOPMENTAL PERSPECTIVE ON SPECIFIC LEARNING DISABILITIES is the third volume in the **Monographs in Developmental Pediatrics** Series.

Other published volumes in this series include:

Primitive Reflex Profile by Arnold J. Capute, M.D., M.P.H., Pasquale J. Accardo, M.D., Eileen P. G. Vining, M.D., James E. Rubenstein, M.D., and Susan Harryman, R. P. T.

The Pediatrician and the Developmentally Delayed Child by Pasquale J. Accardo, M.D., and Arnold J. Capute, M.D., M. P. H.

A NEURODEVELOPMENTAL PERSPECTIVE ON SPECIFIC LEARNING DISABILITIES

Pasquale J. Accardo, M.D.

Assistant Professor of Pediatrics
The Johns Hopkins University
School of Medicine

Developmental Pediatrician
The John F. Kennedy Institute
for Handicapped Children

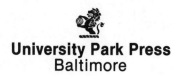

University Park Press
Baltimore

UNIVERSITY PARK PRESS
International Publishers in Science, Medicine, and Education
233 East Redwood Street
Baltimore, Maryland 21202

Copyright © 1980 by University Park Press

Composed by University Park Press, Typesetting Division.
Manufactured in the United States of America by
The Maple Press Company.

Library of Congress Cataloging in Publication Data

Accardo, Pasquale J.
A neurodevelopmental perspective on specific learning
disabilities.
(Monographs in developmental pediatrics; v. 3)
Bibliography: p.
Includes index.
1. Learning disabilities. 2. Developmental neurology. I. Title.
II. Series. [DNLM: 1. Learning disorders.
W1 M0567LP v. 3 / WS1110 A169n]
RJ496.L4A22   371.9   80-12302
ISBN 0-8391-1590-3

Contents

Preface

> But what has been said once, can always be repeated.
>
> Zeno of Elea

> Do not fear to repeat what has already been said. Men need [the truth] dinned into their ears many times and from all sides.
>
> René Laënnec

> Everything that needs to be said has already been said. But since no one was listening, everything must be said again.
>
> André Gide

> What I tell you three times is true.
>
> Lewis Carroll

The field of learning disabilities is one of great confusion for all involved—the children, their parents, and various professionals. A wise pediatrician once said that when the experts in a field are themselves confused, then confusion represents the epitome of knowledge. Indeed one is very skeptical of claims to have discovered *the* answer, the secret remedy, the magic pill, the technical miracle that generations of competent workers failed to uncover. The unknowns (perhaps with some unknowables) far outnumber the knowns. This book will be at fault if it fosters the illusion of a clearly demarcated area with lucid signposts; the state of the art is characterized by confusion and ignorance.

Significant advances are slow in coming. In a standard textbook on reading disorders (Bond and Tinker, 1973), approximately two-thirds of the citations are pre-1960, over 40% pre-1950, and about one-quarter pre-1940. A number of older books have endured (e.g., Money, 1962b; 1966a; P. Wender, 1971); even Huey's (1908) seminal work describes surprisingly current concerns. Probably the greatest single advance in the past half-century has been the recognition that no one discipline has the competence to manage the learning-disabled child. Many edited texts outline a team approach to the diagnosis and treatment of such children: Adamson and Adamson (1979), Flower, Gofman, and Lawson (1965), Newton (1978), and Tarnopol (1969a). The present volume focuses exclusively on the pediatrician's role and attempts to provide him with a general introduction to the entire field. (It is like one of the half-dozen blind wise men expostulating on the nature of an elephant.)

Almost every sensory modality has been implicated in the etiology of learning disabilities; perhaps only olfaction and taste have (thus far) been spared the typical uncontrolled study documenting a statistically significant (but clinically meaningless) correlation with learning problems or hyperactivity. Although cognitive models have not yet yielded significant practical benefits (Schroeder, Schroeder, and Davine, 1978), a rationalist (cf. N. Chomsky, 1973) or linguistic approach seems to hold the greatest promise.

There exists a bewildering array of possible treatments: patterning exercises, dietary fads, yoga, alpha wave conditioning; one of the latest methods spins children around until they vomit. "The list is endless as well as exasperating. We must ask ourselves why some of these remedies (so reminiscent of snake oil) become so widely accepted. It is because the voice of the physician is not heard in the land of education. This very silence is taken as approval" (Newton, 1976). Again, "physician involvement is essential to countermand the multitude of cure-alls advocated by cultists preying upon the sensitivity of distraught parents" (Keys, 1977). Some basic assumptions need to be questioned. Werry's insight remains valid: "The area of learning disorders is beginning to resemble past efforts at curing mental retardation, with enthusiasm outrunning both theory and evaluation of therapy. Just because learning-disabled children are of normal intelligence does not mean that their deficit of learning is necessarily any more treatable than general learning disability (that is, mental retardation)" (Menkes and Schain, 1971).

In the first edition of *Drug Evaluations,* the AMA Council on Drugs (1971) was courageous enough to characterize many drugs as "irrational"; consider the pathos with which future generations will look back on our present folly if we lack a Weyer to fit that most appropriate epithet to even the more accepted therapeutic modalities in the field of learning disabilities. Sufficient outcome studies exist to suggest that the emperor has no clothes.

Though "inconclusive, trivial or sadly incomplete" (Rourke, 1975), the vast learning disability literature does reflect some measure of clinical insight, which ought not be discarded for theoretically interesting but unproved novelties. The present handling of this literature may sometimes recall the style of Eriugena, who often resorted to authority in support of heterodox positions.[1]

The use of global diagnostic categories, such as minimal brain dysfunction (MBD) and specific learning disability (SLD), is analogous to the use of "cerebral palsy" to encompass a heterogeneous group of motor disorders with a common factor—a central nervous system etiology. If one employs a sufficient number of refined tests and measures, it is possible to define any syndrome out of existence (Dykman, Peters, and Ackerman, 1973). Although replacement of the acronyms MBD and SLD by more meaningful terms is devoutly to be wished and finds almost universal support, there is absolutely no agreement on exactly what to substitute for them. Everyone suffers from his own pet classification scheme of unproved utility.

Karl Popper said that science begins with myths and with the criticism of myths; one might add that science continually creates new myths and that the problem of individual differences may very well be exaggerated by our current scientific mythology. Parents and professionals need to be able to tolerate a high degree of uncertainty. The physician who can foster a loving acceptance of the child who paces to a different drummer is not practicing something called advocacy but rather something called pediatrics.

This work was supported in part by Project 917, Maternal and Child Health Service. Figures and line drawings were prepared under the supervision of Mr. Leon Schlossberg. Photographs are by Mr. William Diehl. The prints were prepared for publication by Zuhair Kareem, Chief of Biomedical Photography, and by Raymond E. Lund, R. B. P., F. B. P. A., of Pathology Photography of The Johns Hopkins University. Barbara Kelner, M.L.S., and Jean Dang of the Kennedy Institute Library helped with the references. The handwritten manuscript was reduced to a legible typescript by Judith Brown.

---

[1]E. Gilson, 1955, *History of Christian Philosophy in the Middle Ages*, Random House, New York; cf. J. J. O'Meara, 1969, *Eriugena*, Mercier Press, Cork.

For

Jennifer

who read before kindergarten

Matthew

who refused to read until everyone else did

Claire

who prefers to eat books

and   Patricia

who helped with the reading for this book.

A NEURODEVELOPMENTAL PERSPECTIVE ON SPECIFIC LEARNING DISABILITIES

THE ANALOGICAL CONTEXT

> The doctor said that so-and-so indicated that there
> was so-and-so inside the patient, but if the investiga-
> tion of so-and-so did not confirm this, then he must
> assume that and that. If he assumed that and that,
> then . . . and so on.
>
> Tolstoy
> *The Death of Ivan Ilyich*

Children fail to learn in school for many reasons. Factors such as impaired general health, poor nutrition, frequent truancy (or school absence for other reasons), and sociocultural deprivation may all play a role. Sensory loss (defective vision or hearing) is investigated intensively, found infrequently, and causally associated with childhood learning problems even less frequently. Emotional disturbances are extremely rare in the etiology of learning disabilities but become increasingly more common with age as secondary manifestations of inappropriate class placement and overly high parent/teacher expectations. Of all those children referred for medical evaluation of school failure, the majority fall into the intrinsic or organic group (Table 1). But it must be remembered that the greater part of school underachievers are never referred for such an assessment. There is a preselection of cases to exclude those children with the more obvious environmental etiologies and motivational problems. When such a child is referred for pediatric evaluation, it is usually because someone has noted that he: 1) has normal ability, 2) is trying his best, and yet 3) persists in being unable to learn adequately with the usual teaching methods.

Paine (1962, 1968) described the brain as exhibiting four major areas of dysfunction, each of which in turn could manifest milder variants of disorder: cerebral palsy is a major motor impairment, the choreiform syndrome or the clumsy child syndrome reflect minor motor involvement; mental retardation is a major cognitive impairment, borderline intelligence (the slow learner) reflects minor cognitive involvement; cortical blindness or central auditory imperception is a major sensory impairment, visual-perceptual disabilities reflect minor sensory involvement; a convulsive disorder is a major electrical impairment, subclinical epilepsy (an abnormal EEG without clinical seizures) reflects minor electrical involvement. The pediatric assessment focuses on these different areas of cerebral function since the cognitive and motor

Table 1. Etiologic factors in a clinic population

Extrinsic (Environmental)		Intrinsic (Organic)	
General	Specific	General	Specific
Sociocultural deprivation, 15%–50%	Emotional block, 1°:1% 2°:25%–90%	MBD, 75%	Dyslexia, 5%

The extrinsic/intrinsic dimensions refer to cause; the general/specific dimensions to effect; the diagnostic labels are examples of entities commonly occurring in each category. This division is not exclusive, and the figures will vary a great deal depending on the nature of the physician's referral practice, the utility of his reports to the multidisciplinary evaluation, and the sensitivity of local teachers to an organic contribution to learning problems.

symptoms of gross brain damage syndromes like mental retardation and cerebral palsy are mirrored in the milder signs associated with minimal brain dysfunction (MBD) (Table 2). The physician's contribution to the multidisciplinary evaluation is to view the child as occupying a point somewhere on the spectrum of chronic neurological handicaps (Figure 1). A careful investigation for evidence of organic involvement should not, however, be taken to imply that *all* cases of school problems with *some* signs of minor neurological dysfunction are, therefore, completely biologically determined; it should, rather, indicate an attempt to give appropriate weight to nonenvironmental causal factors.

While there remains much confusion over diagnostic labels, a basic underlying agreement on the concept of learning disability

Table 2. Brain dysfunction syndromes

	Mental retardation	Cerebral palsy	MBD
Perinatal risk factors	+	+	±
Genetic component	+	−	±
Irritable/colicky infant	−	+	±
Language delay	+ +	−	±
Dysarticulation	−	+	±
Gross neurological findings	±	+ +	−
Soft neurological findings	±	+ +	+
Abnormal EEG	+ +	+ + +	+
Subscore scatter	±	+ +	+
Perceptual deficits	±	+ +	+
Hyperactivity/short attention span	±	+ +	+
Cognitive deficit	+ + +	+ +	+

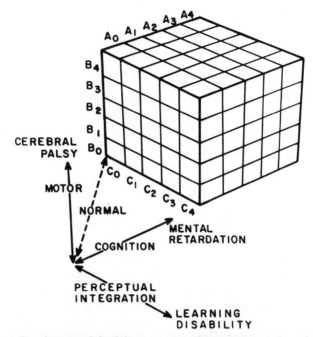

Figure 1. Developmental disabilities matrix. Although the number of variables could easily be multiplied to produce an n-dimensional figure, this cubic matrix allows one to approximate the interrelationships among the various developmental disabilities. A fourth dimension (time) is obligatory: the matrix should be visualized as a plastic structure that demonstrates slight distortions in shape as it moves to the right. The location of various chronic neurologic conditions on the matrix may be illustrated by the following examples: $A_0B_0C_0$=normal child; $A_4B_4C_4$=severely retarded, severely motor impaired child with significant perceptual dysfunction; $A_3B_0C_0$=moderate global retardation with no motor disability or perceptual dysfunction; $A_0B_2C_1$=mild cerebral palsy with normal intelligence and minimal perceptual dysfunction; $A_0B_0C_4$=severe dyslexic with normal intelligence and no soft neurologic signs; $A_0B_1C_3$=MBD child with normal intelligence, "clumsy child" syndrome, and moderate perceptual dysfunction; $A_3B_0C_4$=moderate retardation with severe central communication disorder ("autistic" child). (From Accardo and Capute, 1979.)

has been documented (Vaughan and Hodges, 1973). A generally accepted definition of learning disability is lacking, but it appears that most professionals do share a fair degree of common ground once their technical jargon is translated. The extremely large number of terms used to describe children with learning problems reflects different concepts of etiology and symptom primacy. Psychoneurological (D. J. Johnson and Myklebust, 1967) or neurological learning disability (L. B. Silver, 1971b) probably best characterizes children whose general intellectual function is normal but certain of whose cognitive processes are impaired secondary to brain dysfunction. The child with a significant neurological contribution to his learning problem is called a specific learning disability (SLD).

Attempts to divide SLD children into discrete subgroups have not been very successful. Denckla (1972) found that only 30% of such children fit into specific categories (15% dyslexic syndrome, 10% dyscontrol syndrome, and 5% Gerstmann syndrome), with the other 70% representing a mixture. Owen et al. (1971) defined five groups, into which only 42% of their subjects could be placed without overlap. Thus, although relief from the confusion of global terms would seem to lie in the direction of specific syndrome identification, effective subclassification has hardly begun.

Whether the SLD is secondary to brain damage (the continuum of reproductive casualty), brain dysfunction, such as congenital hypoamphetaminemia (P. Wender, 1971), a biological variant (Werry et al., 1972) made prominent by societal expectations or some other hypothesized etiology, the academic delay is frequently interpreted as a maturational lag. These children's learning and behavior can certainly be attributed to uneven development of cortical functions (de Hirsch, Jansky, and Langford, 1966; Kinsbourne, 1973a; Satz and van Nostrand, 1973), but the misleading aspect of the term *maturational lag* lies in its implication of later catch-up within a predictably short time period (cf. Denhoff, Hainsworth, and Siqueland, 1968). In reality, such "catch-up" is an illusion of perspective. If one uses tests appropriate to early school-age children, the older SLD child will no longer demonstrate the errors characteristic of younger neurologically impaired children; but he will exhibit a persistance of his learning problem when the assessment is geared to age-appropriate cognitive tasks. For example, of learning-disabled children receiving a special class placement (1.5% of the total school population), only one in four was able to be mainstreamed within 5 years. Although they made 1.1 years of reading progress in their first year of special education, this rate dropped to 0.5 years by their fourth year to give them an overall gain of 2.9 years over 4 years (Koppitz, 1971). Those children with fairly mild degrees of impairment may nevertheless benefit from starting school (or at least reading) at a later age, but their ability to integrate well into a regular class after a few years reflects more the wide heterogeneity of grade levels than any resolution of their deficit (cf. Snyder, 1979).

Table 3. Minimal brain syndromes

	Clumsy child	Dyslexic	MBD
Family history	±	+ +	+
Perinatal factors	+	−	+ +
Speech delay	±	+ +	+
Dysarticulation	±	−	+ +
Behavioral symptoms	+	−	+ +
IQ	Normal	Normal, ↑	Normal, ↓
V-P discrepancy	V > > P	P > > V	P > V, V > P, V = P
Subscore scatter	+	±	+ +
Perceptual-motor deficits	+ +	±	+ +
Soft neurological signs	+	−	+ +
Response to medication	−	−	+ +

With very little supportive evidence, the clumsy child has been considered to represent right (or nondominant) hemispheric involvement, the dyslexic child left (or dominant) hemispheric damage, and the MBD child bilateral or diffuse brain damage dysfunction (cf. Hartlage, 1979; Peters et al., 1973).

MBD

Because of its attempt to encompass just about every variety of minor neurological involvement, the term *minimal brain dysfunction* (MBD) has been the source of "maximal neurologic confusion" (Gomez, 1967). The MBD syndrome complex classically includes hyperactivity, distractibility, short attention span (SAS), impulsivity, poor motor coordination, general clumsiness, and specific learning disability (cf. Table 3). It is unfortunate that MBD has become identified with its secondary behavioral manifestations (especially hyperactivity) when the critical (and probably primary) component is a learning disability that is in many (but not all) cases associated with an attentional deficit and multiple derivative psychological symptoms. The behavioral signs include emotional immaturity and shallowness, low self-esteem, stubbornness, temper tantrums, fear of being unloved, manipulative and attention-seeking behavior, anhedonia (decreased experience of pleasure and pain), mood lability (a Jeckyll and Hyde character), and social ineptitude (Kinsbourne and Caplan, 1979; P. Wender, 1971). Enuresis may be more frequent in certain MBD subgroups, but the association is not general (Schain and Reynard, 1975; Stewart et al., 1966); Kolvin, MacKeith, and Meadow (1973) noted that enuresis related positively only to reading retardation in girls. In infancy MBD may be suspected by feeding and

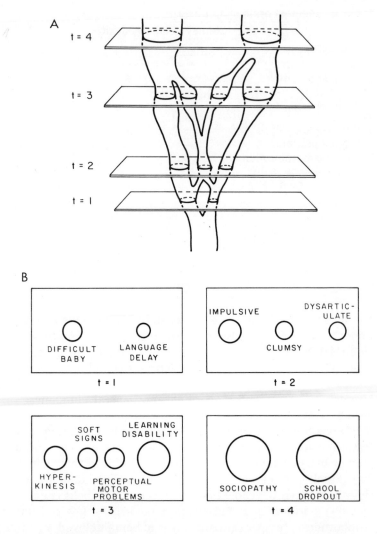

Figure 2. The frequently used Venn diagrams are too abstract to adequately reflect the behavioral reality of MBD. When the temporal variable is excluded, symptoms that may actually be developmentally related appear to be discontinuous. Figure 2A attempts to demonstrate some of the complex interrelationships. When followed over time, this child exhibits rather distinct clinical presentations (B). In infancy (t=1) the baby is noted to be colicky with delayed vocalizations. As a preschooler (t=2) he is impulsive and clumsy, and his early language delay has matured into a mild articulation problem. During the early years of school (t=3), he demonstrates hyperactivity, minor neurological abnormalities, perceptual-motor disturbances, and some degree of learning problems. In adolescence and adulthood (t=4) he may drop out of school and/or display antisocial behavior.

sleeping problems, poor health in the first year, delayed speech, and colic (Bernstein, Page, and Janicki, 1974; Stewart et al., 1966). Of those children who are suspected of being developmentally delayed or cerebral palsied in the first year of life and who are considered normal by 3 years of age, approximately one-third later develop MBD (Denhoff, 1973b). Minimal diagnostic criteria for MBD have never been defined, and there are no universally accepted unique identifying signs. This absence of pathognomonic findings is not uncommon in medicine; the diagnosis derives from the entire complex temporal pattern of symptoms (cf. Figure 2).

The various MBD problem areas of attention deficit, cognitive difficulties, communication disorders, motor incoordination, perceptual-motor disturbances, dyspraxias, emotional immaturity and psychopathy, history of perinatal stress factors, and EEG abnormalities are rarely found together in a single child and do not generally have very consistent relationships with one another (Werry, 1968b). Lucas, Rodin, and Simson (1965) reported that minor neurological abnormalities were more common with a chief complaint of hyperactivity but infrequent with reading disabilities; coordination problems and neurological correlates were associated with a history of obstetrical difficulties or infant feeding problems (especially colic). Denhoff (1973b) noted that the two-thirds of MBD children with hyperactivity have a higher incidence of low birth weight and secondary emotional disorders, whereas the one-third without hyperactivity were more clumsy, more intelligent, and more right-left disoriented. Another way of subdividing MBD children is by the pattern of response to intervention (e.g., drugs) (Figure 3).

The utility of including all of these heterogeneous subgroups under a single rubric can certainly be questioned. In the absence of a generally accepted subclassification system, there are two alternatives: 1) to avoid any diagnostic label and simply describe the strengths and weaknesses of each particular child from as many viewpoints as is practical, or 2) to use a global term like MBD/SLD, recognize its limitations, and supplement it with the same description as in (1). The employment of the acronymic shorthand has been criticized as implying a diagnostic or etiological accuracy where none exists; unfortunately, as is discussed later, the assumed superiority of the descriptive approach turns out to be deceptive. Given the strong historical tendency of the entire field of learning disabilities (whether the perspective is educa-

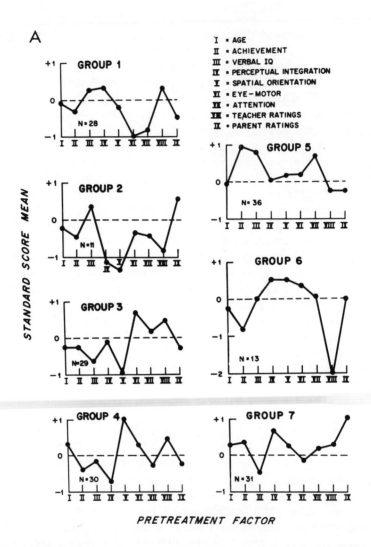

Figure 3. Pattern analysis of response to stimulant medication. Computer analysis revealed seven distinct subgroups with their own pre- and posttreatment profiles. Thus Group 1 demonstrated significant problems with visuomotor tasks and attention before treatment; medication affected the former but not the latter. In contrast, Group 5 presented with isolated conduct disturbances and showed no re-

tional, psychological, or medical) to progress in circles, it would be the height of absurdity to discard along with the term *MBD* its initial conceptual advance—the awareness of a significant organic

B

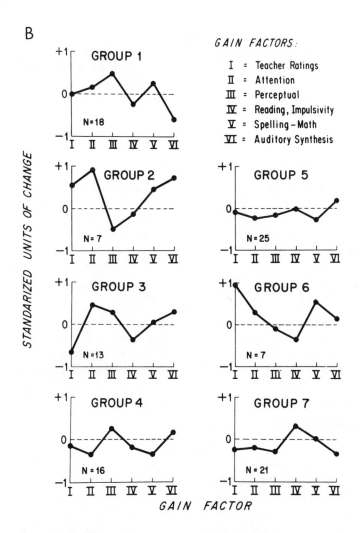

GAIN FACTORS:

I = Teacher Ratings
II = Attention
III = Perceptual
IV = Reading, Impulsivity
V = Spelling – Math
VI = Auditory Synthesis

sponse to medication at all. (Several of the groups were also characterized by marked hemispheric asymmetry on visual-evoked response: Groups 1, 6, and 7, L < R; Group 4, L > R.) (Reprinted from C. K. Conners, Psychological effects of stimulant drugs in children with minimal brain dysfunction, *Pediatrics 49,* pp. 702–708, © American Academy of Pediatrics 1972, with permission.)

contribution to disorders of learning and behavior in children. Reference to MBD (brain damage or brain dysfunction) can be useful in two ways: 1) it defines the medical focus on a developmental disability paradigm in which MBD/SLD includes several minimal cerebral palsy syndromes (Wigglesworth, 1961, 1963) and 2) it alerts the rest of the interdisciplinary team to the biological substrate of these disorders (M. D. Hertzig, Bortner, and Birch, 1969). The evidence to support an association between organic brain dysfunction and the heterogeneous MBD/SLD syndromes is reviewed in later sections of this book.

DYSLEXIA

The very existence of a specific type of learning disability involving reading achievement exclusively has been debated with little agreement over definition or incidence (cf. Rutter, 1969). Eisenberg (1966a) attempted an operational definition of specific reading disability as a failure to learn to read with normal proficiency despite conventional instruction, a culturally adequate home, proper motivation, intact senses, normal intelligence, and freedom from other gross defects. Rabinovitch distinguished three possible etiologies for such reading disability:

1. Brain damage—a neurological deficit akin to aphasia
2. Primary reading retardation—an endogenous developmental lag depending on uneven growth of cognitive processes
3. Secondary reading retardation—an exogenous emotional disturbance (Rabinovitch, 1962; Rabinovitch et al., 1956; Rabinovitch and Ingram, 1962)

Mattis, French, and Rapin (1975) described three distinct dyslexic syndromes:

1. A language disorder with the verbal IQ significantly lower than the performance IQ
2. A buccal-lingual dyspraxia with disarticulation, discoordination, and no verbal-performance IQ discrepancy
3. A visual-perceptual disorder with the performance IQ significantly lower than the verbal IQ

Boder (1971, 1973, 1976) used reading and spelling patterns to delineate three other dyslexic syndromes:

1. Dysphonetic—a primary deficiency in symbol-sound interpretation so that the child's word analysis skills (phonetics) are impaired and his spelling errors are nonphonetic; the reading these children achieve is a global or gestalt function.

Table 4. Two-group theory of reading underachievement

	Reading backwardness	Specific reading retardation
IQ	Low-normal	Normal
♂:♀	1:1	3:1
Family history	+	+
Low socioeconomic status	+	−
Language delay/speech impairment	+	+
Gross neurological problem	±	−
Soft neurological signs	+ +	+
Reading/spelling progress	Poor	Very poor
Math progress	Poor	Fair

Reading-backward children are 28 or more months behind in reading attainment for chronological age; children with specific reading retardation were at least 28 months behind in reading for both age and intelligence. After Yule (1973) and Rutter and Yule (1975).

2. Dyseidetic—these children cannot perceive whole-word gestalts, and their misspellings are phonetic rather than bizarre; they learn to read by phonetics.
3. Dysphonetic and dyseidetic—virtually alexic.

The clinical utility of these last two classifications remains to be proved; evidence is later reviewed to suggest that it is extremely limited.

The main advantage to distinguishing specific reading retardation (dyslexia) from reading backwardness relates to the clinical impression that such "specifics" have a much worse prognosis for ultimate reading attainment than do those children whose reading underachievement is part of a more general learning disability or lowered intelligence level (Ingram, Mason, and Blackburn, 1970). With a 17% overall incidence of reading retardation, 4% of the population does fit a distinct hump at the lower end of the distribution curve (Rutter, 1969; Yule, 1973; Table 4). These specifics also exhibit significantly lower adult reading attainment levels: Rutter and Yule (1975) and Rutter et al. (1976) reported an average reading age of 9 years at 14.5 years of age, less than two-thirds of normal in these "dyslexic" subjects.

INCIDENCE

Lack of agreement over definitions leads to further confusion over prevalence rates. Minskoff (1973) quoted the following figures:

MBD, 5%; two or more grades behind academically, 28%; learning disability or reading disorder, 15%; specific learning disability, 7.5%. In a survey of 2,400 children, J. H. Meier (1971) reported a 20% incidence of learning disabilities and a 4% incidence of hyperactivity. Bax and Whitmore (1973) noted that 6% of school entrants exhibited significant neurodevelopmental disorders; R. G. Miller, Palkes, and Stewart (1973) found a similar 5.5% prevalence rate. The number of children actually receiving some kind of special help from the school system, on the other hand, accounts for a significantly smaller part of the student population— between 1.4% and 1.5% of school children (Koppitz, 1971; Silverman and Metz, 1973).

Although literacy is a major goal of the educational system, literacy rates do not necessarily reflect the prevalence of reading disorders; even severe dyslexics may achieve functional literacy (cf. Appendix B). Because of differences in definition and epidemiological methods, many of the following statistics for reading disability more accurately define some degree of illiteracy. Japan reports the lowest rate of reading problems, less than 1%; Sweden has a prevalence of 8%; Argentina, 12%–14%; Denmark, 15%–18%; Austria, 22%; and France greater than 25% (Downing, 1973; A. J. Harris, 1970).

Surveying an inner city population of black students, Federici, Sims, and Bashian (1976) found a prevalence rate of 14.8% for learning disabilities; the same instrument yielded a 15% rate for suburban white children.

Social class as an index of environmental deprivation does not appear to make a significant direct impact on learning disability statistics. Kappelman, Kaplan, and Ganter (1969), Kappelman, Luck, and Ganter (1971), and Kappelman, Rosenstein, and Ganter (1972) described a population of disadvantaged children with learning disabilities (mean IQ of 79.7). While less than a quarter of them were considered to have a primary emotional disturbance, 55% were diagnosed as showing signs of an organic learning handicap. The neurological basis for these learning disorders is probably indirectly related to socioeconomic status (SES) through the intermediate variable of quality of medical care (especially for pregnant women). Kealy and McLeon (1976) concluded that there was a difference in the rate of diagnosis of specific learning disabilities in different social classes but not necessarily a different prevalence rate. On the one hand, middle to upper class parents may shop around for a diagnosis of learning disability as preferable to one of slow learner or borderline to mild mental retardation. On the other hand, neurologically impaired, low SES children may never be referred for evaluation, the assumption having been made that their poor academic performance is due to motivational and environmental factors, and their parents will not always realize the possibility of a different explanation for their children's learning problems.

SEX DIFFERENCES

Male predominance in reading disorders is reported for many countries—the United States, England, France, and Sweden; fewer nations exhibit female predominance—Germany, India, and Nigeria (Blom, 1972; Downing, 1973). The proportion of same-sex teachers as well as divergent societal expectations (sex role stereotypes) have been advanced to explain these cross-cultural differences in sex ratio. Other hypotheses proposed include the following:

1. Males exhibit more irregular maturation in diverse areas: perception, bladder control, articulation (cf. Glaser and Clemmens, 1965; Maccoby and Jacklin, 1974; Sapir, 1966).
2. Males are more susceptible to environmental influences, with female development being more genetically buffered; there is greater vulnerability of the male brain to both perinatal asphyxia and postnatal lesions (with resulting persistant alterations of brain monoamine synthesis) (Goldman et al., 1974; Simon and Volicer, 1976).
3. Male thought is described as more field independent, analytic, and convergent, leading to higher skills in spatial tasks and arithmetical reasoning; female thinking is characterized as field dependent, global, and divergent, leading to higher verbal skills (Blom, 1972; cf. Guyer and Friedman, 1975).
4. Earlier and stronger brain lateralization of specialized functions in females facilitates verbal development so that girls perform better on verbal tasks from infancy through college age (cf. L. J. Harris, 1978; Kimura, 1967, 1973; Maccoby and Jacklin, 1974).

This last hypothesis, the influence of sex hormones on the rate of hemispheric localization of function (cf. Levy and Levy, 1978), appears to have the greatest potential to explain the other three theories.

HYPERACTIVITY

It is the duty of the instructor to prevent the child's confusing immobility with good, and activity with evil.

Maria Montessori
The Discovery of the Child

Working with mentally retarded and cerebral palsied children, Strauss and Werner (1942) and Strauss and Lehtinen (1947) attempted to describe general behavioral correlates of brain damage. Subjects with frank brain pathology demonstrated a spectrum of attentional peculiarities ranging from short attention span (SAS) to exaggerated fixation or perseveration; their hypervigilance or forced responsiveness to stimuli led them to be easily distracted by new stimuli. They vacillated between inability to focus on a given task and staying with an activity for an inordinate length of time. They exhibited motor disinhibition or organic driveness, frequently described as hyperactivity or restlessness. In addition to conceptual rigidity, emotional lability is also prominent, with inappropriate outbursts and erratic responses to the same stimulus. This entire symptom complex was later noted to occur in children without frank brain damage, and so the concept of minimal brain dysfunction (MBD) developed. Somewhere in this evolution, the idea of a syndrome disappeared and the entire neuro-behavioral complex was reduced to a single symptom—hyperactivity; the "hyperkinetic impulse disorder" was monosymptomatic (Rie, 1975).

Hyperactivity is a vague, ill-defined symptom with multiple etiologies (Table 5). Nongoal-oriented hyperactivity is both qualitatively and quantitatively atypical, different from the exuberance seen in the normal 2-year-old; this latter physiological hyperactivity usually disappears by 3 years of age. In contrast, the driven hyperactivity of MBD remains until adolescence and can occur either continually or sporadically. The predictability rather than the amount of locomotor activity best describes true hyperactivity (Kalverboer, Touwen, and Prechtl, 1973). Occasionally the developmental history reveals that the fetus was hyperactive in utero. "Situational" hyperactivity is a frequent companion to maternal depression; the child's overactivity is an attempt to attract his mother's attention. Constitutional hyperactivity may either accompany or contribute to learning problems. Of 100 chil-

Table 5. Hyperactivity

Type	Definition	Clinical features	Treatment	Prognosis
Toddler overactivity	Normally high activity of this age—should decrease by 3-4 years of age	Active, curious exploration of environment necessary for development. Decreases as inner control begins	Parent education as to developmental normalcy	Good
Constitutional	Inherent temperament present from birth	Normal genetic variation from quiet child to very active. At extreme can look similar to neurologic; no CNS damage or emotional basis	Counseling to assist family in adapting to child's basic personality; stimulant drugs added only if extreme and if parents are unable to adapt	Good
Neurologic	Organic driven behavior; often "high risk" history; may have abnormal neurologic signs	Continuous, random, purposeless movement worsens in groups; often history of being jittery, hard to hold, feeding and sleep problems in infancy	Medications may help; behavioral intervention and parent counseling	Poor to good

Psychogenic	Emotional disturbance manifested by increase in activity			
Lack of internal controls				
Parental control deficit	Lack of parental love and control resulting in poor development of inner controls	Marked increase in activity may occur if lack of parental attention is severe (maternal deprivation); continuous random, purposeless movement	If mild and early, pediatrician can counsel; if later or severe, referral to mental health resource	Fair if slight deprivation; poor if severe deprivation
Early childhood psychosis	Can't form close relationship needed to develop inner controls	Marked variability from total self-absorption to extreme activity	Refer to mental health resource	Very poor
Excessive demands				
Situational	Unrealistic demands produce emotional tension	Fidgeting, squirming motion; selective occurrence in certain situations	Counseling (some families)	Good
Neurotic	Over time, child puts pressure on self independent of environmental demands	Fidgeting, squirming motions	Refer to mental health resource	Poor to good

From Desmond, Vorderman, and Fisher (1978), who adapted it from Schmitt et al. (1973), which gives some interesting estimates of the proportion of hyperactive children falling into the various types. (Reprinted with permission from Assessment of Learning Competence during the Pediatric Examination, in L. Gluck et al. (eds.), *Current Problems in Pediatrics 8* (8).) Copyright © 1978 by Year Book Medical Publishers, Inc., Chicago.)

dren referred for hyperactivity, Kenny et al. (1971) classified 41 as MBD, 35 as mentally retarded, and 18 as emotionally disturbed; a third of these children had electroencephalographic (EEG) abnormalities and half had neurological abnormalities. Laufer (1973) argued that although hyperkinesis and specific learning disability occur together often enough to cause confusion, they can occur separately. Isolated hyperactivity on an organic basis is, however, probably rare; as Rutter (1977) suggested, disorders of attention and activity result more from cognitive impairment than as direct effects of brain damage. Whereas organic hyperactivity tends to be constant, hyperkinesis associated with decreased intelligence is more related to stressful situations (Kinsbourne, 1973b). Hyperthyroidism should be suspected if hyperactivity appears de novo in late childhood or early adolescence.

Bertrand Russell once remarked that research psychologists tended to see their own national characteristics in the laboratory animals they studied. Except perhaps for a particular strain of hyperkinetic dogs (Corson et al., 1971), spontaneous hyperactivity is rare in the animal kingdom, and animal models for hyperkinesis have had to depend on the experimental production of specific brain lesions to produce the desired behavioral symptoms.

When one starts from hyperactivity, it is easy to show that only minimal evidence supports an organic etiology (Dubey, 1976), and cases may be overdiagnosed by as much as four to one (J. S. Miller, 1978). Some of this confusion results from reliance on secondhand observations by parents and teachers. But this kind of error should only occur when the history stops at the chief complaint of "hyperactivity" or relies exclusively on a formal questionnaire. Informants need to be encouraged to describe specific behaviors and activities, precipitating events and other relevant circumstances; as increasing amounts of detail are required, observer bias will tend to reveal itself.

Rapoport and Benoit (1975) found that home observations of children correlated well with psychological reports and teacher ratings of hyperactivity. Although not in agreement with the Pygmalion effect of teacher expectations (Rosenthal and Jacobson, 1968), Paternite, Loney, and Langhorne (1976) found that the incidence of hyperactivity did not vary with social class. A number of longitudinal studies have concluded that hyperkinesis and its associated symptoms are consistent across time (Campbell, Endman, and Bernfeld, 1977; Huessy and Cohen, 1976); although the hyperactivity may diminish with age, distractibility, emotional immaturity, inability to maintain goals, and low self-esteem persist (Minde et al., 1971).

Chess (1972) evaluated the relationship between brain damage and the following signs: hyperactivity, short attention span, distractibility, mood oscillation, increased impulsivity, and perseveration. Perseveration was the only sign that distinguished brain-damaged children from matched controls, but a cluster of three or more signs was significantly related to the presence of brain damage. In a complex behavioral syndrome, no one sign can carry the diagnosis by itself. Unfortunately this is just the role that has been imposed on hyperactivity, and its failure to support the complex superstructure should not be held against either the existence of organic hyperactivity or the validity of a neurobehavioral approach.

BEHAVIORAL THERAPY

The learning theory approach that is so successful in the research laboratory rarely works as well in the real world of the classroom. When dealing with hyperkinesis, behavioral modalities should certainly be employed as adjuncts to other modes of intervention (K. D. O'Leary et al., 1976). Although Ayllon, Layman, and Kandel (1975) were able to reinforce academic skills, the greatest effects of behavior modification have been on social behavior rather than on attention or school performance (S. G. O'Leary and Pelham, 1978). Most studies of operant procedures to date are either anecdotal case reports or involve a small number of poorly defined subjects (Prout, 1977). The suggestion to replace drug therapy by behavioral therapy is an idealistic theory awaiting proof, not a proved theory awaiting implementation.

As is pointed out in the chapter on psychopharmacology, stimulant medication is almost never sufficient therapy for the MBD/specific learning disability (SLD) child. While drugs may ameliorate the attentional problem and facilitate learning, some form of educational intervention is frequently necessary to enable the child to achieve his potential. Although psychotherapy is rarely beneficial for these children, behavior modification in the form of parent counseling by the physician is frequently quite helpful. More extensive behavioral counseling by a professional psychologist is often not readily available and of questionable cost efficacy (Eisenberg, 1978). The pediatrician who feels uncomfortable or inexpert with such cases is certainly free to refer them to a developmental pediatrician specializing in this area. Except with a few of the more severe cases (and these are best handled in collaboration with a psychologist), most behavioral counseling can be performed during the routine office visits or through phone calls to assess effects of medication and school progress.

Behavioral therapy also runs a risk very similar to that of medication—it too can be used to control undesirable classroom behavior without dealing with the true cause or without seeing the child as an individual (Winet and Wikler, 1972); like stimulants, it requires caution in its application. Physicians, teachers, and all professionals working with children need to be familiar with the techniques of behavior modification while keeping in mind the admonition of Schroeder et al. (1978): "Good teachers are good behaviorists but the reverse is not necessarily true." There is no single panacea for these children—medication, teaching methods, psychological therapies. All aspects of treatment need to be coordinated in a comprehensive program that views the child as a complex whole and has as its goal the increase of the child's ability to function independent of any special intervention.

READING, LITERACY, AND DYSCALCULIA

The three R's of Restraint, Rote Memory and Regurgitation.

E. Howard

The book is the taboo *par excellence.*

Arturo Castiglioni
Adventures of the Mind

READING

What a dangerous activity reading is.

Sylvia Ashton-Warner
Spinster

The idea that some kind of auditory intermediate is necessary to reading is very old. In his treatise *The Teacher,* Augustine wrote:

> What if we find words in writing? Are they words, or are they not correctly to be understood as signs of words? To be a word, it must be uttered in an articulate vocal sound with some meaning; but the voice cannot be perceived by any other sense than hearing. Thus it is that when a word is written a sign is presented to the eyes, and this brings into the mind what pertains to hearing (Colleran, 1950).

One must remember Augustine's surprise at Bishop Ambrose— "When he read, his eyes travelled across the page and his heart sought into the sense, but voice and tongue were silent" (*Confessions vi,* 3)—because silent reading was virtually unknown in the ancient world.

Although he admitted that the final problem of reading is comprehension, Elkonin (1973) defined reading as the translation of its graphic model into the sound form of a word. While most nonbehaviorists would view this description as inadequate to the process of reading (see Figure 4), Elkonin stressed that auditory factors are more important than visual ones. He reported that although the sound discrimination necessary to speech develops easily, the sound analysis skills necessary to reading develop much later in children.

That reading cannot be just automatic sequential decoding— the translation of the "seen word" into the "heard word" (auditory surrogate) or the behaviorist's subvocal speech—is attested to by two lines of evidence. First, reading frequently outstrips all

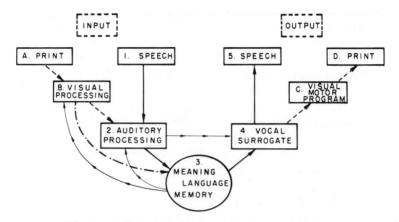

Figure 4. Language processes. 12, auditory perception; 123, reception of spoken language; AB, visual perception; AB 2345, (Immature) oral reading; AB 345, (mature) reading; AB 245, decoding; AB 245 > AB 2345, hyperlexia; 345, expression of spoken language; CD, visual-perceptual motor skills; 45 > 345, "cocktail talk" (in hydrocephalus). AB3 demonstrates a direct route from print to meaning without the mediation of an auditory component; actually much mature reading may still utilize auditory processing. Phonetics and orthography are important in B2, B3, B23, and 4C; semantics and linguistics are important in 23 and 34. The 3 triad indicates the complex cognitive interplay of language (deep structure), meaning (comprehension), and memory (general experience) as reflective of general cognitive level and state of attention. This cognitive complex has a continuous directing influence on visual and auditory processing of language (and other) stimuli: "Meaning leads, and the idea of the whole dominates the parts" (Huey, 1908).

estimates of the decoding potential. Thus, the sequential perception of letters would allow for a maximum reading rate of 35 words per minute when the usual rate is ten times that (Kolers, 1972). G. A. Miller's (1956) magical number of 7 ± 2 as the limit on the mind's ability to process information allows for "chunking," or grouping, data into large units, but the maximal theoretical reading speed still falls short of actual reading achievements by a factor of five (Wolf, 1977). Second, decoding may occasionally be seen to outstrip general reading ability. Silberberg and Silberberg (1967) have described a number of cases of hyperlexia in which word recognition skills were higher than comprehension abilities. Half of their subjects were mentally retarded, autistic, or brain damaged. If this condition is not diagnosed, expectations in other academic areas may be unreasonably high. Interestingly, some of these hyperlexic patients had poorly developed visual and perceptual skills and yet were still able to decode accurately. Guthrie

(1973) noted that while some reading-delayed children had problems with decoding, others appeared to have more specific comprehension difficulties despite adequate sight vocabularies. Reading (in terms of comprehension) seems thus to be surprisingly independent of both decoding and the perceptual processes that decoding may be dependent upon.

The theoretical possibility of purely visual reading was suggested by Huey in 1908. Vernon (1977) agreed that it was possible and Mattingly (1972) considered that some form of it was probable considering that high speed readers were able to go directly to a deep level of language with minimal input. "The meaning seems eventually to leap from the printed page with scarcely any awareness of inner speech" (A. J. Harris, 1970). That an acoustic representation is not needed for a word to be read is supported by data on deaf subjects where such an intermediate is impossible (Gibson, Shurcliff, and Yonas, 1970) and also by observations of phonemic dyslexia; these patients make semantic errors going from the grapheme (written word) to the meaning without passing through the phoneme (e.g., they might read "bird" for "robin") (Saffran and Marin, 1977). It must nevertheless be admitted that much mature reading does involve an auditory component. This will be less true for scientific material and skimming and more true for the reading of "literature" (e.g., poetry). Thus, C. S. Lewis's (1961) "good reading is always aural as well as visual" depends on the nature of the material and the purpose of the reading.

While these points are true for mature, rapid reading, they are less applicable to the beginning reader. The young child usually masters decoding with a great deal of help from acoustic intermediates (cf. Doehring, 1976). As he gets older, he will learn to "chunk" material—to read words faster than letters, and sentences faster than words—to generate hypotheses concerning the meaning of a pattern of symbols and then to sample the text just enough to verify his hypothesis (Kolers, 1972). Reading is a cognitive activity, and "the end product of a cognitive activity is not a bit of verbal behavior but a deep cognitive structure" (Neisser, 1967). This constructive aspect of reading allows Goodman (1967) to characterize it as a "psycholinguistic guessing game"; in many ways it does resemble the process of piecing together a solution to the Sunday *Times* crossword puzzle. Even blind persons engage in this type of sampling: when reading Braille, the right hand examines the general outline of the words and is followed by the left hand, which glides over only a part of the letters; a variable amount of material is left for conjecture (Huey, 1908; cf. Kimura, 1973).

Although blindness does not prevent the effective use of spoken language, deafness severely impedes the mastery of written language (F. S. Cooper, 1972). Furth (1971) characterized the deaf as linguistically deficient: in the absence of mental retardation they achieve an average reading level short of grade three, and hardly 10% get above grade four. Blind children's reading competence is much closer to their intelligence level (Fraiberg, 1977). The sensory deprivations apparently exert their effects through their impact on language.

Languages with more regular orthography do seem to give rise to lower incidences of reading disability (Downing, 1973). But to blame English orthography for the high rate of dyslexia in English-speaking countries is not entirely satisfactory. First, the relation of conventional English orthography to the sound structure of English is closer than is usually thought (and is probably getting closer). Second, the nonphonetic aspects of English orthography are motivated rather than arbitrary; they represent deeper levels than the merely phonetic (C. Chomsky, 1970; cf. Jespersen, 1956). The most regular orthography (*pace* Bernard Shaw; cf. Edwards, 1969) is not necessarily the most efficient.

Ideographs avoid the problems of letter-sound associations. Whereas phonemic symbols are more complex and abstract at the beginning, once mastered, they allow a greater number of potential combinations; ideographs, on the other hand, are easier at the beginning and have similarities to both numerals and the token and sign languages being taught to nonhuman primates. Japanese offers the combination of an ideographic script (Kanji) with a phonetic syllabary (Kana) (Sakamoto and Makita, 1973) (see Figure 5). Makita (1968) reported a very low incidence of reading disability in Japan—less than 1%—and attributed it to the orthographic regularity of Kana. D. D. Steinberg and Yamada (1978) questioned the results and the interpretations of Makita's questionnaire survey. They found that Kanji ideographs were more easily learned despite being graphically more complex, and they concluded that meaning was much more important than perceptual features. Rozin, Poritsky, and Sotsky (1971) confirmed that ideographs were more easily learned even by inner city reading-retarded American children. C. L. Kline and Lee (1972) studied a

DIFFERENCE OF CHARACTERISTICS BETWEEN ALPHABET AND KANA SCRIPT

ALPHABET		KANA SCRIPT	
LETTER	SOUND	LETTER	SOUND
a	[a][e][ei]	い *	[i]
b	[b] or silent	ろ	[ro]
c	[k][s]	は	[ha]
d	[d][t]	に	[ni]
⋮		⋮	
a consonant or a vowel		a syllable a combination of a consonant and a vowel with which the uttering ends.	
SOUND	REPRESENTATION	SOUND	REPRESENTATION
[f]	f, ph, gh,	na **	な
[f][v]		ni	に
[f] or silent		nu	ぬ
[n]	n kn, gn	ne	ね
[ai]	ais ay, aye, ei, eigh, eye, i, ie, igh, y, ye,	no	の
direct link of 2 or more consonants.		no direct link of consonants. consonants are always linked through a vowel or vowels	
Unstable script-phonetic relationship: every sound IS NOT represented by corresponding specific letter.		Stable script-phonetic relationship: every sound IS represented by corresponding specific letter. *(like in I. T. A.)*	

Figure 5. Difference of characteristics between alphabet and Kana script. The phonetic nature of the Kana script has been thought to explain the very low incidence of reading disability in Japan. (From K. Makita, The rarity of reading disability in Japanese children, *American Journal of Orthopsychiatry 38,* pp. 599–614, © 1968, American Orthopsychiatric Association, Inc. Reproduced by permission.)

population of children bilingual for English and Chinese; the incidence of reading disability was 3% for English (phonetic/auditory/left hemisphere), 5% for Chinese (ideographic/visual/right hemisphere), and 2% for both (mixed), with a 10:1 male predominance in all groups. These results suggest that neither the eye nor the ear (nor one hemisphere) determines the presence of a reading disorder.

LITERACY

> The man who does not read good books has no advantage over the man who can't read them.
>
> Mark Twain

College graduates now comprise 25% of the total labor force. Over the past 20 years the proportion of professionals in the American population has risen 4% while the proportion of blue collar and farm workers dropped by more than 3% each (Ginzberg, 1979). On the one hand, the more menial jobs are being eliminated by automation, and on the other hand, the remaining positions have increasingly inflated academic (namely, reading) requirements. Thus the reading level necessary to survive economically in modern society is slowly but steadily rising.

Educators distinguish three levels of reading skill: 1) the independent level is the highest reading grade at which a child reads easily and fluently without assistance; 2) the instructional level is the highest grade at which a child can read satisfactorily with assistance (i.e., in a classroom); and 3) the frustration level is the lowest grade at which a child's reading skills break down so that he misses at least half the material (Critchley, 1970; A. J. Harris, 1970; Newbrough and Kelly, 1962). The independent level is sometimes also referred to as the functional level. However, functional literacy is the level of ability to read and write that is normally expected of literate people in the area of culture involved (Gray, 1955). Functional literacy is usually defined in relation to the ability to secure appropriate employment (Resnick and Resnick, 1977). A fourth grade reading level or better is expected achievement for mildly retarded persons; the U.S. Census Bureau defines literacy as the completion of 6 years of schooling. An army cook needs at least a seventh grade reading level (Sticht et al., 1972). More recent estimates of the minimum level of reading ability needed in today's world ("technological literacy") range from 8th to 12th grade (Downing, 1973). When one compares these grade levels to the mean scores for high school graduates in a given community, it must be remembered that half the students are functioning below their class mean.

DYSCALCULIA

There is no goodness in mathematics.

Thomas Aquinas, *ST* I, q16 a14

. . .and then the different branches of Arithmetic—Ambition, Distraction, Uglification and Derision

Lewis Carroll

While a mathematics grade level consonant with the child's chronological age, school experience, and intelligence is commonly found in young children with reading retardation, the converse, a specific delay in arithmetic (dyscalculia) with a normal reading level, appears to be encountered more rarely. This may be because of lower expectations for universal mathematical competence (as opposed to literacy) or to a lesser dependence of elementary arithmetic on verbal skills. Many children with reading problems who have been doing better in mathematics start to have more difficulty in arithmetic between third and fourth grades, when "word problems" (requiring reading skills) become more common. Cohn (1971) suggested that basic mathematics was more easily acquired than other symbolic operations (i.e., reading) because of the highly specific relationship between the written symbols and their respective operations. Numerals (representing set functions) may be considered to act very much like Chinese ideographs, with no dependence on phonic associations. Thus, to obtain a reasonable facility with arithmetic, no specialized training would be needed outside of drill and repetition. Problems with the Bender-Gestalt figures have particular significance for mathematics performance (Koppitz, 1963). On the other hand, the multiplication of three-digit by two-digit numbers represents a more complex use of symbols, and difficulties with this kind of problem (e.g., incorrect serial order) would probably reflect more pervasive language (higher order) dysfunctions (Cohn, 1961). More primitive deficits, such as forgetting to carry or failing to recognize the operational symbol (e.g., doing addition instead of the indicated subtraction), are usually part of a more general learning problem, with associated abnormalities of attention and memory. Finally, Cohn (1968) has emphasized the phenomenon of class adherence: no matter how severely involved the individual child is with dyslexia or dyscalculia, the errors exhibited will almost always operate within the appropriate class of letters or numbers. Thus, even bizarre misspellings will not include numerals, and irrational arithmetical solutions will not display letters. When this class adherence is violated (e.g., 1+1=D), then psychogenic factors should be considered.

Pure dyscalculia, defined as a mathematics quotient below 75 in a child without a general learning disability, may not be that rare. Kosc (1974) reported a 6% incidence in Eastern European school children; this is as high as any estimate of specific reading disorders. Kosc also found a genetic predisposition to dyscalculia, and Guay and McDaniel (1977) noted a positive correlation between spatial ability and mathematics achievement. Many of the cases included in these studies may represent forms of the Gerstmann syndrome, which is secondary to parietal lobe pathology: finger agnosia, right-left disorientation, acalculia, and agraphia (Gerstmann, 1940). Some patients with this syndrome also demonstrate constructive apraxia, impaired color perception, and disturbed equilibrium; reading is only insignificantly affected. Clumsiness and dysgraphia are frequently noted in dyscalculic children, and Kinsbourne and Warrington (1963c, d) have developed tests of finger sense for use with children. The questionable concept of a *developmental* Gerstmann syndrome has been employed by Kinsbourne and Warrington (1963a, b, 1964) to distinguish: 1) parietal lobe types of learning disorders (right hemisphere) with poor penmanship and spelling errors that involve incorrect letter sequencing from 2) aphasic types of learning disorders (left hemisphere) with dysarticulation and spelling errors that involve extraneous letters. Applications of the Gerstmann syndrome concept to children must still be considered highly speculative.

The "new math" frequently impresses parents as something out of Lewis Carroll's Looking Glass world:

> "What's one and one and one and one and one and one and one and one and one and one?"
> "I don't know," said Alice, "I lost count."
> "She can't do addition," said the Red Queen.

Piaget, Inhelder, and Szeminska (1960) did demonstrate that children acquire topological concepts before projective geometry ones, with Euclidian intuitions coming last. The new math misapplied this conception and, by introducing set theory before addition, ignored a more basic developmental postulate that the concrete precedes the abstract. M. Kline (1974) chronicled the seriocomic evolution of the new math fiasco, which essentially involved ivory tower theorizing being applied in the classroom in the complete absence of data on how children actually learn arithmetic. Brainerd (1973) later distinguished three processes in the acquisition of number competence: 1) cardination, or set matching, 2) ordination, or sequential quantification, and 3) competence in manipulating natural numbers, or number drill. The "old math" or Pythagorean approach placed primary emphasis on rote drill; the new math stressed cardination or set theory as the best introduction to mathematics. In reality, the invariant developmental sequence is ordination→number drill→cardination. In other words, the new math had completely inverted the optimal order. Even where mixed approaches to the teaching of arithmetic have been employed, the new math has influenced the very vocabulary used in elementary workbooks; thus, terminology from set and number theory makes the reading grade (based on syllables per 100 words; see Appendix A) of a typical third grade workbook approach a college level.

> We expect our children to possess by pubescence a numerical competence much higher than that of an educated Greek or Roman adult of two millenia ago. We have even gone so far as to devise labels that imply mental turpitude on the part of those otherwise normal children who fail to attain the standards of numerical competence that we deem desirable (Brainerd, 1973).

This criticism is only partially correct. There do appear to be children with a specific disability in mathematics that is independent of uninspired teaching. The definition, epidemiology, subclassification, and remediation of this disorder are recorded on pages that are almost blank.

THE NEUROLOGICAL SUBSTRATE

It is a very myopic medical science which works backward from the morgue rather than forward from the cradle.

E. A. Hooton
Apes, Men, and Morons

But it would be . . . quite wrong, to argue: that because I may or must, for certain limited purposes, treat this as if it were that; therefore I am assuming, or have even shown, that this just is that—and that's that.

A. G. N. Flew
Crime or Disease?

The classic neurological approach to disorders of learning and language is rooted in the aphasiological context (Critchley, 1970). In this model, discrete lesions in the adult brain produce fairly specific patterns of expressive and/or receptive linguistic disability (Table 6; Figure 6). For example, in Wernicke's aphasia, the primary auditory receptive area is damaged so that spontaneous speech is fluent (with paraphasias and logorrhea that the speaker is unaware of) but comprehension (of the speech of others), repetition, and naming are all impaired.

Aphasias in childhood have been associated with head trauma, hemiplegia (Byers and McLean, 1962), and temporal lobe seizure foci (Gascon et al., 1973; Shoumaker et al., 1974); those secondary to subclinical seizures are actually composed of three distinct subgroups, all with a generally poor language prognosis (Deonna et al., 1977). But the skills necessary for literacy are not isomorphic biologically with those required for general linguistic competence (Kershner, 1977), and apart from some hints of the progress of hemispheric specialization in childhood, adult aphasia models are not very rewarding in the study of learning disorders.

It is generally accepted that the major or dominant hemisphere (usually the left) is concerned with spoken language, with a mode of information processing that can be described as logical, analytic, serial, or sequential; the minor or nondominant hemisphere (usually the right) is more concerned with total patterns, and its more diffuse mode of information processing may be char-

Table 6. Types of aphasia

Type	Speech fluency	Compre- hension	Repetition	Lesion
Broca (motor)	− [a]	+	−	Posterior inferior frontal
Wernicke (sensory)	+ [b]	−	−	Posterior superior temporal
Conduction	+	+	−	Arcuate fasciculus
Isolation	+	−	+	Association cortex
Anomic	+	+	+	Angular gyrus

Adapted from Geschwind (1972) and Hardin and Merson (1974); cf. Luria (1965).

[a] − Impaired, limited.

[b] + Intact.

acterized as holistic, gestalt, synthetic, spatial, or geometrical (Kimura, 1967, 1973). Speech lateralization to the dominant hemisphere occurs earlier in females, but nondominant specialization is prominent in males by 6 years of age and in females by 13 years of age (Witelson, 1976). If a bilateral representation of spatial processing persists for too long, this overdevelopment of traditionally right hemispheric functions could exert a crowding effect on language ability localization—what Witelson (1977) has hypothesized as "two right hemispheres, none left."

NEUROANATOMY

Almost a century ago, Hinshelwood (1917) associated the angular gyrus of the dominant hemisphere with congenital word blindness, but Hermann (1959), in reviewing autopsy material, found no evidence for central nervous system pathology in dyslexics. Geschwind (1962, 1965, 1968, 1972) postulated the left angular gyrus as a possible substrate for dyslexia; functionally, area 39 links visual and auditory stimuli, a process essential in reading. The entire inferior parietal lobule (which includes the angular gyrus) is known to mature very late cytoarchitectonically, with its

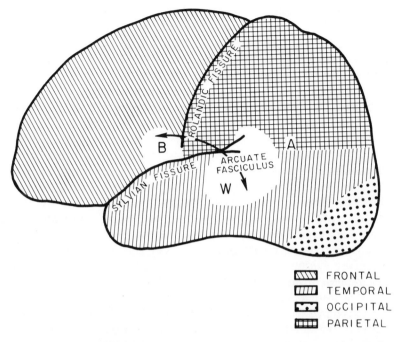

FRONTAL
TEMPORAL
OCCIPITAL
PARIETAL

Figure 6. Types of aphasia. B, Broca's area; W, Wernicke's area; A, angular gyrus. (After Penfield and Roberts, 1959.)

development often not being complete until the end of childhood. In the temporal speech region, the area behind Heschl's gyrus (area 41, the primary auditory cortex), the planum temporale, is grossly larger on the left side in the majority of autopsy specimens; this enlargement of the planum temporale (which contains a significant portion of Wernicke's area) accounts for the greater length of the left Sylvian fissure and larger size of the left temporal lobe (Benson and Geschwind, 1968; Geschwind and Levitsky, 1968). This asymmetry of the temporal lobes is apparent between 29 and 31 weeks of gestation, with the left side being larger and the right side evidencing greater gyral complexity (Chi, Dooling, and Gilles, 1977; Galaburda et al., 1978). A reversal of the usual asymmetry (with the right side larger than the left) can be observed on a computerized tomography (CT) scan in some dyslexic children (Hier et al., 1978), and there may be a sexual dimorphism in the distribution of these reverse asymmetries (cf. Witelson, 1976) to help explain the predominance of males in all types of learning disorders.

Lesions in a variety of cerebral loci are capable of producing hyperkinesis in different experimental animals. The frontal and prefrontal association areas (8–12) yield fairly marked hyperactivity (Kennard, Spencer, and Fountain, 1941; Shetty, 1973), with Walker's area 13 being the extreme point for maximal motoric stimulation (Livingston et al., 1947; Ruch and Shenkin, 1943). Damage to the interpeduncular nucleus (Bailey and David, 1942), the caudate nucleus (G. D. David, 1958), the ventromedial nucleus of the hypothalamus (Wheatley, 1944), and a variety of other rostral hypothalamic areas (Maire and Patton, 1954) produce hyperkinesis less consistently. Striatal injury hyperactivity is more dependent on external stimuli (Mettler and Mettler, 1942). Hyperkinesis secondary to parietal lobe lesions is not as marked as that due to frontal damage (Beach, 1941). In general, the frontal regions of the brain (along with the other areas mentioned above) are considered to exert an inhibiting effect on the ascending reticular activating system (RAS) (Magoun, 1963). The RAS is concerned with general arousal and orienting to novel and habituation to repeated stimuli. Although discrete frontal lesions lead to hyperkinesis, extensive frontal damage produces a frontal lobe syndrome of passivity, inertia, and lack of motivation and critical attitude (Chalfant and Scheffelin, 1969; Luria, 1973). The prefrontal regions most significant in the control of hyperkinesis mature rather late, usually between 4 and 7 years of age (Luria, 1973).

Radiation in utero, carbon monoxide poisoning, and direct pallidal lesions affect markedly different brain areas and yet produce very similar pictures of hyperactivity (Norton, Mullenix, and Culver, 1976). Hyperactivity would appear to be a final common behavioral pathway to express many distinct and overlapping disturbances in the modulation of lower centers by higher ones (cf. the concept of diencephalic dysfunction in Laufer and Denhoff, 1957, and Laufer, Denhoff, and Rubin, 1954). Finally, the actual anatomical destruction of tissue is not necessary; a pharmocological lesion of dopamine pathways with intracisternal 6-hydroxydopamine (60HDA) produces in rat pups permanent reduction in the levels of brain dopamine and a hyperactivity that responds to amphetamine therapy (Shaywitz et al., 1976; Shaywitz, Yager, and Klopper, 1976; Shaywitz, Cohen, and Shaywitz, 1978; Sorenson, Vayer, and Goldberg, 1977). Although the hyperkinesis abates with age, the rats exhibit persistent learning disabilities as adults. Neurochemical lesions may be as effective as structural abnormalities in the production of disorders of behavior and learning.

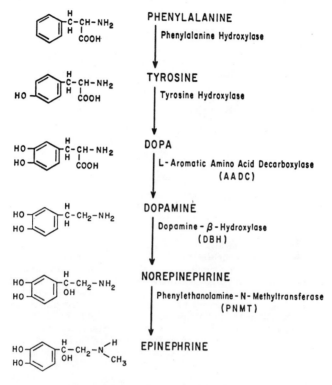

PHENYLALANINE

Phenylalanine Hydroxylase

TYROSINE

Tyrosine Hydroxylase

DOPA

L-Aromatic Amino Acid Decarboxylase (AADC)

DOPAMINE

Dopamine - β - Hydroxylase (DBH)

NOREPINEPHRINE

Phenylethanolamine - N - Methyltransferase (PNMT)

EPINEPHRINE

Figure 7. Synthetic pathway of catecholamines. (From D. J. Cohen and J. G. Young, Neurochemistry and child psychiatry, *Journal of the American Academy of Child Psychiatry 16,* pp. 353–411, ©1977, with permission.)

NEUROCHEMISTRY

Two groups of biogenic amines have been implicated as central neurotransmitters: the indoleamines and the catecholamines. Studies on platelet levels of the indoleamine serotonin have been inconclusive; a major role for serotonin metabolism in the symptomatology of minimal brain dysfunction (MBD) is doubtful. Research on catecholamines like dopamine and norepinephrine has been more extensive and has documented a number of possible explanations for the origin of symptoms and for the understanding of the efficacy of stimulant treatment (Shaywitz, Cohen, and Shaywitz, 1978). Catecholamine synthesis is presented in Figure 7; the principal degradation product of dopamine is homovanillic acid (HVA), whereas norepinephrine breaks down to vanillylman-

DOPAMINE

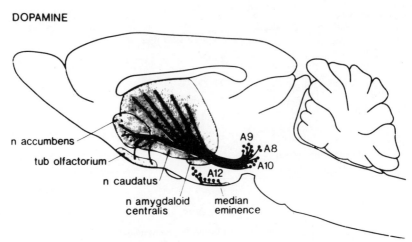

Figure 8. Dopaminergic pathways. A longitudinal section along the midline of the rat brain demonstrates the three major dopaminergic tracts, with the principal nerve terminal regions being indicated by shading. The nigrostriatal pathway goes from the substantia nigra (A8, A9) to the caudate and amygdaloid nuclei. The mesolimbic pathway ascends from the interpeduncular nucleus (A10) to the nucleus accumbens and the olfactory tubercle. The tuberoinfundibular pathway stays completely within the hypothalamus, crossing from the arcuate nucleus (A12) to the median eminence. (From U. Ungerstedt, Stereotaxic mapping of the monamine pathways in the rat brain, *Acta Physiologica Scandinavica 367*(suppl.), pp. 1–48, ©1971, with permission.) Cf. Lindvall and Björklund (1974).

delic acid (VMA) and 3-methoxy-4-hydroxy-phenylethyleneglycol (MHPG). Although biochemically dopamine is a precursor of norepinephrine, the tracts that produce dopamine (dopaminergic pathways, Figure 8) are anatomically and functionally distinct from those utilizing norepinephrine as a neurotransmitter (noradrenergic pathways, Figure 9) (J. R. Cooper, Bloom, and Roth, 1974). The three dopamine pathways are fairly discrete: 1) the nigrostriatal tract is concerned with motor function; it is this functional unit that is affected in Parkinson's disease; 2) the tuberoinfundibular tract regulates the synthesis and secretion of trophic hormones within the hypothalamic-pituitary axis; and 3) the mesolimbic tract is involved with those behavioral functions that respond to amphetamine therapy (S. H. Snyder and Meyerhoff, 1973). The two ascending noradrenergic pathways are more diffuse, with their nuclei more caudally located and their nerve terminations creating a larger collateral network than the dopamine tracts (Figures 8, 9, 10); this widespread radiation is in keeping

NORADRENALINE

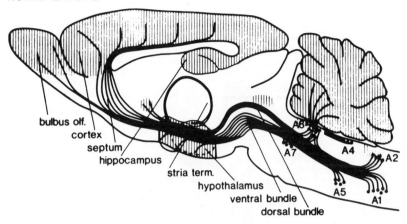

Figure 9.   Noradrenergic pathways. The two ascending noradrenaline tracts are shown in this midline longitudinal section through the rat brain, with the principal nerve terminal regions being indicated by shading. The dorsal tract ascends from the locus coeruleus (A6) to the cerebral cortex, cerebellar cortex, and hippocampus. The ventral ascending tract has cell bodies throughout the pons and medulla oblongata with connections to the hypothalamus, limbic system, and lower brainstem. (Two descending noradrenergic pathways, not illustrated, innervate the spinal cord and regulate blood pressure.) (From U. Ungerstedt, Stereotaxic mapping of the monoamine pathways in the rat brain, *Acta Physiologica Scandinavica 367*(suppl.), pp. 1–48, ©1971, with permission.) Cf. Lindvall and Björklund (1974).

with these systems' function of modulating emotional states and moods (D. J. Cohen and Young, 1977; Moskowitz and Wurtman, 1975). All the catecholamine tracts overlap with one another and with the median forebrain bundle, which is the reward center of the brain (Olds, 1962; Routtenberg, 1978; L. B. Silver, 1971b); the ventral norepinephrine pathway is probably the most closely enmeshed in this pleasure center and has been identified as the localization site for the euphoriant action of stimulant drugs (S. H. Snyder and Meyerhoff, 1973).

Shaywitz, Cohen, and Bowers (1977) demonstrated decreased levels of HVA in cerebrospinal fluid in MBD children; there were no differences in the levels of 5-hydroxyindoleacetic acid (5-HIAA), the principal metabolite of serotonin. They hypothesized a reduced turnover of brain dopamine as somehow involved in the etiology of MBD. Shetty and Chase (1976) found no differences in HVA or 5-HIAA between MBD and control children, but amphetamine administration decreased HVA levels in the MBD

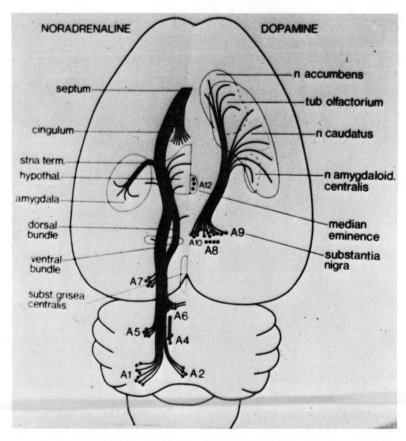

Figure 10. Catecholamine pathways. Horizontal section through rat brain illustrates the ascending dopamine and norepinephrine tracts. The noradrenergic system has its nuclei more caudally located, but its terminations are much more diffuse than those of the dopaminergic system. (From U. Ungerstedt, Stereotaxic mapping of the monoamine pathways in the rat brain, *Acta Physiologica Scandinavica 367* (suppl.), pp. 1–48, © 1971, with permission.) Cf. Lindvall and Björklund (1974).

population. Similarly, Shekim et al. (1979) reported that dextro amphetamine lowered MHPG (a norepinephrine metabolite) excretion in drug responders.

Neurotransmitter physiology in humans is still in its infancy. The implication of the nigrostriatal and mesolimbic dopaminergic pathways and the ventral noradrenergic tract in the pathogenesis is still circumstantial. The impressive technology necessary to document these early results should not blind the clinician to their fundamental ambivalence. Alterations in biogenic amine metabolism provide an organic substrate for problems of learning and behavior, but such alterations may themselves result from earlier environmental influences (Axelrod et al., 1970; Eleftheriou and Boehlke, 1967).

BRAIN DAMAGE

Whether lesions are structural or biochemical, the localization of such defects is not the same as the localization of a function (Zangwill, 1963). The identified loci are necessary but not sufficient conditions for specific behaviors; in Gregory's (1974) phrase, the brain is too like porridge. Analogies from animal to human loci do not always hold: spatial memory in rodents is located in the hippocampus; in man, in the parietal lobe (Olton, 1977). Difficulties with "neurometric phrenology" suggest some truth to Lashley's (1963) law of mass action in which the quantity of equipotential cortex damaged is more significant than its location.

The correlation between the progression of symptoms and the evolution of brain lesions is relatively poor. Asphyxia in monkeys may produce extensive brain damage but only transient hard neurological signs; adaptive behaviors will be delayed but memory and learning tend to be permanently impaired to some degree (Sechzer, Faro, and Windle, 1973). In the chronic recovery stage, the lesions are encephaloclastic; as the behavior improves over time, the brain pathology actually extends into regions originally unaffected (Towbin, 1971; Windle, 1968).

According to Luria's (1973) law of hierarchical structure of cortical zones and Vygotsky's (1962) theory of dynamic localization, brain lesions in early childhood have a systematic effect on higher cortical processes, whereas involvement of the same region in adults predominently influences lower functions; the interaction between damaged and intact brain structures is from below upward in the child and from above downward in the adult. The adult's ability to compensate for the permanent loss of neural tissue is facilitated by resorting to the use of higher cortical functions, such as language (Luria, 1963). A partial restoration of function through an internal reorganization and transfer to higher (i.e., more conscious) levels of function is probably the preferred mode of treatment even in children (cf. Luria, 1961). That any structuring of sensory input at an automatic level will bring about the required higher cortical synthesis is both unproved and unlikely.

ETIOLOGY

The potency of a cause is greater, the more remote
the effects to which it extends.

Aquinas,
C.G. III, C, 87

EMOTIONAL DISORDERS

A quarter of a century ago, when emotional disturbance was considered a common cause of learning disabilities, the psychogenic
literature consisted mainly of anecdotal case reports (Natchez,
1968, Part I, Section A; Weil, 1970). Heller (1963) observed that
the kinds of emotional disorders found in poor readers were indistinguishable from the emotional disturbances of normal readers.
Thus, there was no specific psychiatric diagnosis that made a
child more susceptible to reading problems. Rabinovitch (1962),
who had proposed the concept of a secondary or exogenous reading retardation characterized by anxiety, negativism, depression,
psychosis, and emotional blocks, confessed that over the years he
had come to view the incidence of such secondary reading retardation as much lower than first anticipated (Rabinovitch and
Ingram, 1962). Blanchard (1946), a strong proponent of the psychoanalytic viewpoint, estimated that only 20% of children with
reading disabilities had significant emotional problems. Rutter
(1974) concluded that emotional disturbance did not play an important part in the etiology of specific reading retardation;
psychotherapy has little effect on reading proficiency (Schiffman,
1962). After reviewing the various concepts of Freudian plumbing
as applied to learning disability, Kurlander and Colodny (1969)
suggested that theories reflecting a constitutional cognitive disorder were much more reasonable. Primary emotional disturbance
as a cause of learning disability is now considered extremely rare
(Bakwin and Bakwin, 1948; Clements and Peters, 1962; R. D.
Snyder and Mortimer, 1969). Unfortunately, in the training of
teachers the emotional basis of learning and its disorders is still
given priority to the exclusion from consideration of constitutional and organic factors.

When one starts with school children diagnosed as emotionally disturbed, careful evaluation demonstrates that 40% of such
children have cognitive or perceptual-motor disorders (E. Z.
Rubin and Braun, 1968). Instead of emotional disturbances caus-

ing learning disabilities, the reverse appears closer to the truth: there is a significant constitutional, hereditary, or physiological basis for many behavioral disorders of childhood, and this organic substrate is most clearly reflected in the cognitive dysfunction (J. L. Orton, 1966; Salk, 1973). If the pediatrician completely removed psychogenic factors from consideration as etiologically significant in cases of specific learning disability, he would rarely be in error.

GENETICS

Specific reading disability has long been considered to have a strong genetic component. In his series of dyslexics, Hallgren (1950) reported that 88% had a history of reading problems in one or more members of their immediate family, with 40% to 60% of the parents being involved; he postulated a Mendelian dominant mode of inheritance. Drew (1956) suggested a similar genetic mechanism for congenital word blindness, a parietal lobe deficit that produces a disturbance in gestalt function similar to that produced by the Gerstmann syndrome. Bakwin (1973) studied reading disability in twins and found a 29% concordance in fraternal twins and an 84% concordance in identical twins. Mattis et al. (1975) noted 79% positive family histories in dyslexic children with no signs of brain damage.

Learning-disabled children had a 30% to 40% incidence of learning disabilities in family members who had no history of perinatal stress (L. B. Silver, 1971a). Owen et al. (1971) found that many parents of learning-disabled children still had symptoms of learning disabilities themselves; the child's Wechsler Intelligence Scales for Children (WISC) discrepancies tended to be marked when the parental history was positive. The Scot clans of Campbell and Maclean demonstrate a clustering of delayed speech, specific difficulties in reading and writing, and ambidexterity or poorly developed handedness (Ingram, 1963).

Hyperactivity appears to be more common in siblings (Welner et al., 1977; P. Wender, 1972) and blood relatives (J. Morrison and Stewart, 1974); there is a high concordance for hyperactivity in monozygotic twins (Willerman, 1973). For children in foster placement, there is a 50% rate of hyperactivity in full siblings of index cases, but only a 10% rate for their half-siblings (Safer, 1973; cf.

J. Morrison and Stewart, 1973, on adopted hyperactive children). The families of hyperactive children show a clustering of alcoholism, hysteria, and sociopathy, along with a history of hyperactivity in the childhoods of parents, aunts, and uncles (Cantwell, 1972; J. Morrison and Stewart, 1971). The absence of an increased incidence of depression in these families confirms the impression that hyperkinesis is not often a form of manic-depressive illness (Stewart and Morrison, 1973). The strength of the correlations in the above reports support a significant genetic contribution to the heterogeneous components of the minimal brain dysfunction (MBD) syndrome (cf. Omenn, 1973).

Gross chromosomal defects (such as the aneuploidy in trisomy 21) usually cause significant mental retardation in addition to multiple organ system involvement. Klinefelter syndrome (47XXY) and the 47XYY tall males tend to have lower IQs as well as speech and language difficulties (Walzer and Richmond, 1973; Witkin et al., 1976). Turner syndrome (45X0), with the short female habitus, exhibits deficits in space-form perception, visuoconstructional recognition, copying the Bender forms, the draw-a-person test, and arithmetic (Money and Alexander, 1966). Waber (1979) found that Turner females were poor on word fluency, right-left perception, visual-motor coordination, and motor learning; rather than evidencing a specific deficit in spatial ability or an exaggerated "female" profile, these deficits were interpreted as weaknesses in all those areas in which male or females were known to have group superiority. Despite their severe spatial deficits, patients with Turner syndrome rarely exhibit reading problems. Hyperactive children have normal karyotypes (Warren et al., 1971), so this test is not warranted without other indications. There is no known technique for the prenatal diagnosis of childhood problems of behavior and learning.

PERINATAL FACTORS

In general, the incidence of mental retardation, learning disabilities, and reading disorders is higher in children with perinatal insults, such as anoxia (Jordan, 1964). More specifically, the relationship between reading disability and perinatal complications is significant but of a low order; more studies support than fail to support the association (Balow, Rubin, and Rosen, 1975). For example, Kawi and Pasamanick (1958) related reading disorders in children to maternal preeclampsia, hypertensive disease, and bleeding during pregnancy. Rhesus incompatibility, on the other hand, does not lead to an increased incidence of reading disability when intelligence and deafness are controlled (Walker et al., 1974).

Millichap et al. (1968) noted that 57% of hyperkinetic children had a history compatible with brain damage occurring during pregnancy. But the increased incidence of bleeding, toxemia, hypertension, low birth weight, convulsions, trauma, unconsciousness, anoxia, and irritability was not as striking when records were reviewed and controls utilized; the only factors that still appeared significant were an abnormally short or prolonged labor and the use of forceps (Minde, Webb, and Sykes, 1968). Several studies suggest an association between MBD/specific learning disability (SLD) and birth order, with an increased incidence in first- or second-born children (Dykman et al., 1973; Laufer and Denhoff, 1957). In a longitudinal study, Werner and Smith (1977) advanced evidence to support a concept of double vulnerability: children with severe perinatal stress factors tended to have poor long-term outcomes, but for those with only moderate perinatal stress factors the long-term outcome depended more on the quality of the environment (i.e., the ability of the parents to respond appropriately to a child with an impaired biological disposition).

Of all perinatal factors, *prematurity* has been the most intensively studied. Meier (1971) reported a 20% rate of prematurity in a learning-disabled population compared to 5% in controls; surveying a population of MBD children, Bernstein et al. (1974) found a 72% incidence of pre- or perinatal complications, with a prematurity rate of 15% being the most frequent (control incidence of 7.5%). Evidence has remained fairly consistent over several decades that when premature babies grow up they do worse than term babies in intelligence level and academic achievement (Bjerre and Hansen, 1976; Corrigan et al., 1967; Knobloch, Rider, and Harper, 1956; G. Wiener et al., 1965). Males are more vulnerable than females and the babies with the lowest birth weights seem to be the more severely affected (R. A. Rubin, Rosenblatt, and Balow, 1973). It must be remembered that the incidence of complications of prematurity varies indirectly with birth weight. For babies with the same low birth weight, there is still some debate over whether the true premature (weight appropriate for gestational age, AGA) does better than the small-for-dates infant (weight small for gestational age, SGA) (cf. Neligan et al., 1976); the evidence seems to be shifting toward a worse prognosis for the SGA, or intrauterine growth-retarded (IUGR), babies. Fitzhardinge and Steven (1972) followed a population of small-for-dates infants and reported the following complications: MBD in one-quarter, abnormal electroencephalograms (EEGs) in two-thirds, speech defect in one-quarter to one-third, and poor school performance in one-third to one-half; males had consistently worse outcomes. These results were attributed to diffuse mild brain damage.

The *fetal alcohol syndrome* of pre- and postnatal growth deficiency (low birth weight, short stature, microcephaly), developmental delay (borderline to mild mental retardation with fine motor clumsiness), small palpebral fissures, and multiple other mild anomalies is secondary to excessive maternal consumption of alcohol during pregnancy (Jones and Smith, 1973, 1975; Jones et al., 1974); many of these cases will present clinically as clumsy, mildly dysmorphic, learning-disabled children. Denson, Nanson, and McWatters (1975) reported a positive correlation between hyperkinesis and maternal smoking during pregnancy. Since heavy maternal smoking is associated with decreased birth weight, the mechanism for affecting later behavior and learning may be one of intrauterine malnutrition. Fetal alcohol babies are also small, but whereas general intrauterine malnutrition may play a role, alcohol appears to exert specific toxic effects on the developing fetus as evidenced by the associated malformations.

NUTRITION AND FOOD ALLERGY

Children severely malnourished in infancy later demonstrate poor school performance and lower IQ scores (S. A. Hertzig et al., 1972). While marasmus is usually considered to be more devastating to brain development than kwashiorkor (cf. Chase, 1973), Richardson, Birch, and Hertzig (1973) were unable to show an association between the age of initial hospitalization for malnutrition (i.e., the first 6 months of life versus the second year of life) and the degree of later impairment. Even relatively brief periods of starvation can have long-term effects: children with pyloric stenosis in infancy had normal IQs, but their learning abilities were negatively correlated with the degree of starvation before pylorotomy (Klein, Forbes, and Nader, 1975). Nutritional status in the first 2 months may be critical for the later development of attention and short-term memory.

Breast-fed babies do consistently better on later reading attainment than do bottle-fed infants (Rodgers, 1978). This phenomenon may be mediated through a prolongation of tyrosinemia with high protein bottle feedings; increased levels of tyrosine produce a small but significant lowering of IQ and perceptual functioning (Menkes, 1977; Menkes et al., 1972).

Feingold (1975a, b) has popularized the notion of an epidemic of hyperactivity and learning disabilities due to increased ingestion of certain low molecular weight chemicals, such as artificial food flavors and colors (especially tartrazine, FD&C yellow #5) and salicylates. (Tartrazine can produce asthma and urticaria in aspirin-sensitive patients according to Juhlin, Michaëlsson, and Zetterström, 1972.) He has also related the ingestion of foodstuffs containing the offending agents to behavior and learning problems in children with mental retardation and petit mal epilepsy and has claimed a 30% to 50% favorable response rate to the Kaiser-Permanente (K-P) diet, which excludes such substances (Feingold, 1976). Response takes about 3 weeks; however, dietary indiscretions show effects within hours and last for days.

Palmer, Rapoport, and Quinn (1975) could find no difference in the consumption of food additives between hyperactives and controls. Brenner (1977) reported a positive effect of the Feingold diet, but could not rule out a placebo effect. C. K. Conners et al. (1976) noted a 25% reduction in hyperkinetic symptoms on the diet. In the study by Goyette et al. (1978) there were no effects on behavior after a challenge dose of artificial food color other than a slight decrease of sustained attention. The more carefully controlled and designed the research, the more subtle the behavioral changes observed; the strongest effects appear to be found in a small subset of preschool children (Harley, Matthews, and Eichman, 1978; Harley et al., 1978). Consistent behavioral changes probably occur in only 2% to 8% of children. Considering: 1) that excluding the salicylates in fruits may lead to a vitamin C deficiency, 2) that the response rate to stimulant medication is much higher, and 3) that the diet works best in that age group where hyperactivity presents little problem and where medication would only rarely be considered, the place of the K-P diet outside of research would appear to be problematical (cf. E. H. Wender, 1977;

Williams et al., 1978). As Spring and Sandoval (1976) suggested, public advocacy has far outstripped the research basis for dietary therapy; such reliance on simplistic solutions and panaceas can only blind us to the more relevant individual differences. (For other reviews, see Bierman and Furukawa, 1978; Palmer, 1978).

Orthomolecular therapy is a related shotgun approach using megavitamins, trace elements, and diet to prevent hypoglycemia (Cott, 1971); Pauling (1970) had popularized one component of this regimen in the treatment of the common cold. The hypoglycemia that these children are supposed to have usually rests on a questionable interpretation of a rather normal looking glucose tolerance test. The whole orthomolecular rationale is derived from an unproved therapeutic modality for schizophrenia; megavitamins for childhood psychosis and learning disabilities are of no value and are potentially toxic (Committee on Nutrition, 1976). Brenner (1979) has suggested an interaction between the level of a trace element (copper) and positive response to the Feingold diet, but at present this must be classed as a "correlation between fuzzies."

It is still unclear whether the untoward effects of Feingold's low molecular weight substances is based on an allergic or toxic mechanism; his use of the term *behavioral toxicology* would suggest the latter. Epidemiologically, children with documented allergic diseases have not been reported to display a higher incidence of specific learning disabilities. Crook (1974a, 1975) and Mayron (1979) have proposed a spectrum for the allergic tension-fatigue syndrome that relates it to the MBD/SLD complex. Allergies, especially to foods, presumably affect the central nervous system to produce a pale, tired, hyperactive, and irritable child. A specific neurological component of the effects of allergens is actually unnecessary; the general symptoms of allergy, such as stuffiness, drowsiness, fatigue, and torpor, would affect classroom performance. Crook (1974b) recommended a stringent elimination diet with slow reintroduction of food classes to identify the offending substances. May (1975) has criticized the concept of the allergic tension-fatigue syndrome as the great masquerader; he views it more as a current crutch and a species of quackery.

The idea of a *rare* child exhibiting MBD/SLD symptomatology secondary to an allergic tension-fatigue syndrome actually seems to make more sense clinically than many of the claims from the Feingold and orthomolecular camps. The paranoia over food additives and the mystique of vitamins seem to be contributing to an increasing medicalization of eating (cf. Szasz, 1974). The philosophy that you are what you eat might more profitably be applied to a study of the effects of different ethnic dishes on the development of national characteristics of thinking and thus contribute to world peace. Given the totally unproved nature of dietary approaches to learning and behavior disorders, there is a fanaticism implicit in most of what is written about this area that insists on ignoring other relevant variables. L. H. Smith (1977) is perhaps the one exception; he attempts to place nutritional speculations within the perspective of the whole child and his family. The potential (and probably small) contribution that diet has for the field of learning disorders is only being obscured and delayed by its overenthusiastic publicists.

LEAD

O. David, Clark, and Voeller (1972) showed that hyperactive children had higher body lead burdens by challenging hyperkinetic patients with a chelating agent. O. J. David et al. (1976) further demonstrated a marked behavioral improvement after chelation therapy had lowered these children's elevated but nontoxic lead levels; those who did not improve with treatment had perinatal and developmental histories more suggestive of a brain damage etiology. Thus lead would appear to be a true example of "behavioral toxicology." But although subclinical intoxication with lead has been implicated in learning disorders and behavior problems of childhood (Needleman, 1973), the specificity of the association is unclear. De la Burdé and Choate (1975) reported striking behavior problems accompanied by lower full scale IQs and poor visual, perceptual, and fine motor coordination; similarly, Landrigan et al. (1975) judged fine motor abilities and WISC-R performance subtests to be the most impaired. On the other hand, Needleman et al. (1979) found the greatest effects of subclinical plumbism to be on the verbal subtests of the WISC-R and on measures of auditory and speech processing; hyperactivity was infrequent but attentional problems severely affected classroom behavior and were dose-related to the original lead burden. The reasons for these discrepancies must await further research, but in the meantime a history of pica (ingestion of nonfood substances) in early childhood should be sought.

The results of animal studies do not particularly clarify the situation. Lead has been reported to produce in rats a hyperactivity that does respond, paradoxically, to stimulant drugs (Silbergeld and Goldberg, 1974); decreases in central dopamine levels have been hypothesized to contribute to an altered norepinephrine-dopamine ratio in the brain (Sauerhoff and Michaelson, 1973). Golter and Michaelson (1975) could not confirm the catecholamine changes.

VISION

Since the time of Hinshelwood, visual factors have played a prominent role in the thinking about reading disability. But the rate of visual defects appears to be the same in good and poor readers (Cassin, 1969; Norn, Rindzuinski, and Skyvsgaard, 1969; Shearer, 1966). When children with serious refractive errors and reading problems are prescribed glasses, their reading rarely improves (L. J. Lawson, 1968). Although the incidence of visual acuity defects was similar in both groups, Eames (1948, 1962) did find that hypermetropia and exophoria were more common in reading failures than in controls. Defects in depth perception and ocular muscle imbalance should not affect reading and are actually more frequent in good readers. *Strabismus* has been identified as a risk factor in learning disorders (Bax and Whitmore, 1973; Charlton, 1972).

The visual system has a strongly topographical organization, with a relatively one-to-one mapping of the optic retina onto the cortical retina (Figure 11). Although the spatial pattern is preserved, a complex analytical system (responsive to specific attributes, such as orientation, movement, and contrast) is applied even at the level of the primary visual receptive area (J. A. Anderson, 1977). The degree to which higher cognitive processes override supposedly primitive visual-perceptual processes (even when the latter are disordered) is perhaps best reflected in the frequency of proofreader's errors.

Critchley (1970) mentioned reports of an increased incidence of *color blindness* using the Ishihara test in dyslexic children as probably not significant. J. D. Cohen (1976) noted that the rate of color blindness depended on the conceptual content of the particular test. Thus Justen and Harth (1976) found that the decreasing

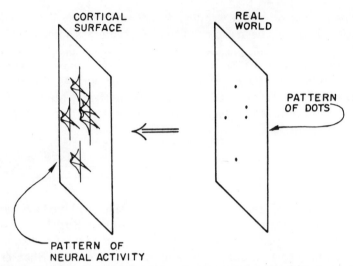

Figure 1. Visual cortical projection. A pattern of dots gives rise to a pattern of activity distributions on the cortical surface; adjacent points on the retina generally map into adjacent points on the primary visual cortex. The spatial pattern of the stimulus is preserved but with fascinating magnifications and distortions. (From J. A. Anderson, in D. La Berge and S. J. Samuels (eds.), *Basic Processes in Reading*, pp. 27–90, © 1977, Lawrence Erlbaum Associates, Inc., Hillsdale, N.J., with permission.)

incidence of color blindness in learning disability with age was secondary to the problems these children had with figure-ground perception—a significant element in most tests for color blindness. A much rarer difficulty with colors was reported by Geschwind and Fusillo (1966): patients with infarctions of the left calcarine cortex and the splenium had problems *naming* colors. Success on a test for color blindness suggests that all the above factors are intact; failure on such a test is open to numerous interpretations.

In uncontrolled studies optometric vision therapy (for an average of 60 hours over a 5-month period) claims a 93% cure rate for learning disorders (W. I. Swanson, 1972). Keogh (1974) found existing efficacy studies to be inadequate and too limited to enable a final judgment. That eye movement control is unrelated to reading ability is suggested by the excellent reading skills of children with congenital nystagmus (L. J. Lawson, 1968). Furthermore, Goldberg and Arnott (1970) demonstrated that abnormalities on the electronystagmograph were actually secondary to the degree of comprehension of the material being read. Visual learning is done by the brain and not by the eye.

Another part of optometric training programs involves disorders of eye dominance. On the one hand, sighting tests used to determine eye dominance are unscientific (Money, 1966b), and on the other hand, the methods employed to change mixed dominance are not neurologically sound (Bettman et al., 1967). The relationship between visual fields and hemispheric dominance needs tests of a much greater refinement than are in clinical use for its demonstration; functionally the two eyes are interchangeable. When S. Orton (1928) compared reading-disabled children having left eye dominance with those having right eye dominance, he could find no difference in their clinical presentations. Since there is no association between ocular dominance or mixed eye-hand preference and reading ability (L. J. Lawson, 1968), there really is not anything to treat. A joint organizational statement of three professional groups concluded that there is no support for visual training (muscle exercises, ocular pursuit, glasses) or neurological organization training (laterality, balance beam, perceptual) (Ad Hoc Committee of AAP et al., 1972; cf. Benton, 1973; Flax, 1973; Keys, 1977). Peripheral eye defects do not produce learning disorders, and optometric training does not improve learning problems. Apart from the unwarranted expense, such training is probably damaging because of the false hope it engenders and the inappropriate focus it places on noneducational remediation.

HEARING

Deafness causes a significant depression of all linguistic functions (Furth, 1971). High frequency deafness is mostly congenital; with the auditory input filtered, the child appears to hear but not to understand (Matkin, 1968). The incidence of high frequency deafness is approximately 4 per 1,000; undetected, these children exhibit poor speech comprehension, behavioral difficulties, and learning failures (with mathematics as poor as reading) (U. M. Anderson, 1967). Even a mild high frequency loss may be disabling to a young child because: 1) consonants have a higher frequency than vowels (Bond and Tinker, 1973), 2) women have higher-pitched voices, and 3) female teachers predominate in the elementary grades.

Chronic otitis media before 2 years of age has been associated with a significant loss of expressive and receptive language skills and auditory discrimination. The long-term effects on reading and mathematics appear to be related to the number of episodes (Holm and Kunze, 1969; Kaplan et al., 1973). Shurin et al. (1979) warned that the relative risk for the persistence of middle ear effusion after an acute otitis media was almost four times as high in children under 2 years of age (and almost three times as high for whites as for blacks). Zinkus, Gottlieb, and Schapiro (1978) used myringotomy between 3 and 5 years of age as an index of the severity of otitis media; they described the resulting learning profile characterized by substantial delays in speech and language, auditory processing deficits (especially auditory sequential memory), disturbances in auditory visual integration, and reading and spelling disorders (with arithmetic less affected) as secondary to a distortion of auditory signals during a critical period. Similarly, Masters and Marsh (1978) documented that a higher percentage of learning-disabled children had a history of middle ear pathology; many of these children passed pure tone audiometry but failed impedance audiometry employing tympanometry. It must be cautioned, however, that some serious questions have been raised over the reliability of tympanometry to assess Eustachian tube function (Siedentop et al., 1978; on hearing tests see Bluestone and Shurin, 1974; Henderson, 1975).

Inferior performance on auditory discrimination has been noted in children with reading disorders (Flower, 1965). But Blank (1968) showed that while retarded readers failed to discriminate pairs of similar-sounding words and repeated pairs of such words poorly, they had no problem repeating the words singly. Their primary difficulty appeared to be more one of attention and memory than perceptual discrimination. As usual, failure has many interpretations, and higher-order processes are more important than more elementary ones.

In attempting to identify a subgroup of learning-disabled children whose learning problems are secondary to a fluctuating hearing loss in early childhood, the critical factor that is frequently ignored is the possibility of chance overlap. Thus children with documented aphasia often have a high frequency loss (Merklein and Briskey, 1962). Eisenson (1969) described the typical audiological report on an aphasic child as identifying a degree of hearing loss insufficient to explain the severity of the observed language impairment. Do the reported hearing losses cause the central auditory processing disorders, or do they represent chance associations that, however, accentuate a preexisting cortical dysfunction? Further epidemiological research will help to answer this question. Whatever the order of the relationship, otitis media will continue to receive appropriate medical therapy.

VESTIBULAR DYSFUNCTION

Frank and Levinson (1973) claimed that dyslexia was secondary to dysfunction of cerebellar-vestibular circuits; lesions in this pathway would interfere with the eye's ability to scan letters and numbers sequentially. They found that subclinical nystagmus by electronystagmography could distinguish dyslexics and that "cerebellar-vestibular harmonizing agents," such as cyclizine (Marezine), cured 97% of reading disorders. (Clinical studies establishing safety and efficacy of Marezine in children have not been done.) Similarly, de Quiros (1976) characterized a large segment of the learning-disabled population as suffering from vestibular disorders. Vestibular hyporeflexia by caloric stimulation supposedly reflects restlessness from internal stimuli, motor coordination problems, and difficulties in controlling skilled eye movements. Ayres (1978) has identified a subgroup of learning-disabled children with hyporeactive nystagmus to a rotational stimulus; this group reportedly exhibits greater academic gains in response to therapy that enhances the processing of vestibular input than those children with hyperreactive responses (cf. M. Steinberg and Rendle-Short, 1977). Rapin (1974) warned that with children under 10 years of age there would be at least a 25% disagreement between clinical tests of vestibular dysfunction and electronystagmographic findings. Keating (1979) compared the Southern California Postrotatory Nystagmus Test with electronystagmography and concluded that the observer impressions in the former were completely unreliable in learning-disabled children. The evaluation of therapeutic efficacy of modes of treatment based on such unreliable instruments is an exercise in futility. At this point it is needless to comment that the impressive neurological-sounding theories that underpin these approaches are on the order of wild speculations.

SEIZURES AND ANTICONVULSANTS

Approximately 10% of children with learning disabilities have seizures as compared to 1% of the general population (Hart et al.,

1974; cf. J. H. Meier, 1971). On the other hand, the school performances of two-thirds of children with epilepsy are significantly worse than those of nonepileptic children (Stores, 1978). Since the old concept of reading epilepsy has been pretty much discarded (cf. Forster, 1975), poor seizure control or the not infrequently related brain damage probably accounts for most of this association. Febrile seizures by themselves lower later performance on psychological measures but not on achievement tests (Schiottz-Christensen and Bruhn, 1973); the incidence of mental retardation in the febrile convulsion population is 8%, with girls more vulnerable to later disability (Wallace and Cull, 1979).

Left (or dominant) hemisphere spikes on the EEG in boys have been related to reading retardation as well as to decreased attention and hyperactivity (Fedio and Mirsky, 1969; Stores, 1978). Treating subclinical seizures with anticonvulsant medication, such as diphenylhydantoin, however, may actually lower reading performance (Stores, 1978; Stores and Hart, 1976); ethosuximide (Zarontin) has been shown to depress verbal comprehension and memory in children being treated for petit mal epilepsy (Guey et al., 1967). Phenobarbital prophylaxis for febrile convulsions often aggravates hyperkinesis in the preschool child; its long-term effects on learning are unknown. Anticonvulsants are toxic agents with numerous side effects; their potentially adverse effect on learning and attention needs to qualify any tendency to overprescribe them. Anticonvulsants should be used to treat seizure disorders, not learning disorders. (Cf. section entitled Other Drugs.)

HEAD INJURY

Only a third of children with serious head injuries develop any kind of posttraumatic syndrome; this is much lower than the incidence after head injury in adults. Males, as expected, appear to be more vulnerable. About a fifth of children with head trauma develop behavioral symptoms, the most common being hyperkinesis, decreased attention span, difficulty controlling anger, and headache (Black et al., 1969).

INFECTIONS

The TORCH group of infections (toxoplasmosis, rubella, cytomegalovirus, herpes) and other bacterial and viral meningitides and encephalitides frequently have devastating effects on the brain, but milder cases of these infections as well as clinically less well defined agents (Sells, Carpenter, and Ray, 1975) may cause later behavioral and cognitive disorders. Silent cytomegalovirus infections, for example, produce a school failure rate approximately three times normal and in excess of that secondary to hearing loss (Hanshaw et al., 1976). Measles (rubeola), German measles (rubella), chickenpox (varicella), or mumps before the age of 3 years (especially around the age of 2 in males) have been related to specific delays in reading and mathematics in later childhood (Wagenheim, 1959). Presumably, at certain ages the brain is more vulnerable to the effects of these viruses. Coxsackie B4 viral infection in infant mice has been shown to persistently impair brain catecholamine metabolism (Lycke and Roos, 1975).

DEGENERATIVE CONDITIONS

The clinical presentation of most central nervous system degenerative disorders in childhood will rarely be confused with MBD/SLD; the developmental history is often the most important feature in the differential diagnosis. Wilson's disease (hepatolenticular degeneration) is a rare autosomal-recessive condition that usually presents with liver disease and no neurological symptoms. Occasionally clumsiness, dysgraphia, tremors, slurred speech, and behavior disorders may be noted late in grade school; the absence of any of these symptoms throughout the first half of school should suggest the possibility of a degenerative process. A careful search for hepatic signs and Keiser-Fleischer rings should be made (cf. Sass-Kortsak, 1975). This is a treatable disease; the copper accumulation in liver, brain, kidney and cornea responds to D-penicillamine.

MISCELLANEOUS

Ott (1976) proposed that hyperactivity and learning disabilities were secondary to the radiation stress condition of fluorescent lights; he reported dramatic improvements following the placing of lead shields over the cathode ends of the fluorescent tubes. Occult endocrine causes are rarely implicated in learning disabilities. G. E. Park and Schneider (1975) noted elevated thyroxine levels in dyslexic children; Tiwary et al. (1975) found that synthetic thyroid-releasing hormone (TRH) significantly improved the behavior of MBD children. Replications of these studies are lacking, the mechanisms implicated are unclear, and their overall significance is dubious.

PERCEPTION
AND LANGUAGE

I saw more with my mind than with my eyes.

Christy Brown
My Left Foot

Chief Justice. I thinke you are falne into the disease:
For you heare not what I say to you.
Falstaff: Very well, my Lord, very well: rather an't
please you, it is the disease of not Listning, the mal-
ady of not Marking, that I am troubled withall.

Shakespeare,
The Second Part of *King Henry IV*

For sensation itself is but vision nascent, not the
cause of intelligence, but intelligence itself revealed
as an earlier power in the process of self-construc-
tion.

Coleridge
Biographia Literaria

Perception as a modality of etiology, diagnosis, and treatment has
been predominant in the field of learning disabilities for many
more years than either research or outcome data warrant. Most
of the schools of thought (loosely categorized as "perceptual")
reviewed in the present chapter support their theories with elaborate but very questionable interpretations of neurological functioning; since most of the intended audience is nonmedical, neuro-
physiological oversimplifications and inaccuracies get overlooked
amid a welter of half-digested neuroanatomical jargon. To those
who judge scientific merit by the weight of its terminology rather
than the accuracy of its content, such speculations must appear
impressive indeed.

Frostig and Orpet (1969) distinguished two kinds of perception: in the narrow sense perception is concerned with the recognition and discrimination of stimuli; in the wider sense perception
gives meaning to events and objects. They claimed that both were
necessary, but that if perception (narrow sense) were faulty, then
perception (wider sense) would also be disordered. It may be truer
to reverse this and suggest that perception in the wider sense actually controls perception in the narrow sense. Thus Kohler (1964)
found that by using special prismatic eyeglasses, the world would

appear to be upside down for only a short time, and the experimental subjects' brains would soon correct the perceptual distortion. There is an increasing body of experimental data to suggest that perception and conceptualization are not sequential but reciprocal (Vellutino et al., 1977); that is, perception appears to partake of the nature of thought and is not easily (if at all) isolated from processes called cognitive. Thus Gregory (1974) characterized perceptions as guesses—hypotheses—about what object stimulated the nerves; indeed, the act of perception seems to have all the strengths and weaknesses of the process of syndrome formation.

Piaget (1969) listed 14 differences between intelligence and perception; he stressed that perception was limited to the here and now and could not select what was necessary, whereas intelligence in some way always exceeded the data. Nevertheless, he admitted that perception prefigures operational notions. Through a series of experiments, Bryant (1974) demonstrated that infants and young children depend heavily on logical inferences to make most of their perceptual judgments; in reinterpreting many previous studies of perception he showed that memory had been ignored as a critical variable. One must be cautious not to objectify the step between sensation and conceptualization into an independent entity; as Pièron (1945) observed, sensation itself is highly symbolic.

Perceptual-motor theories assume that specific (both quantitative and qualitative) experiences are critical to the development of higher cognitive processes. They frequently cite Piaget's stage theory in support of their speculations (cf. Phillips, 1969). Wolff (1969) criticized these misinterpretations of Piaget: normal children exhibit variable strategies to achieve the stage of logical thought; children with severe sensory deficits use alternative pathways to arrive at grossly the same view of the physical world. Since the perceptual deficits of motor-impaired children are not usually related to their motor disability but rather to the attendant brain damage, a program to normalize their perceptual-motor experiences would seem to be an exercise in futility. Thus thalidomide children with variable degrees of phocomelia (shortened or absent limbs) actually exhibit performance IQs *higher* than verbal IQs (McFie and Robertson, 1973). In cerebral palsy one does not find equivalent degrees of perceptual impairment with right and left hemiplegics; right-sided brain damage affects perception to a much greater extent (Wedell, 1960).

Over 10 years ago Werry (1968a) commented that the "efflorescence of the nonmedical professionals offering 'perceptual motor training' should be viewed with a skepticism proper to all new treatment methods until scientifically impeccable data attest to its value." The remainder of this chapter offers for consideration: 1) that the data are in, 2) that skepticism is no longer appropriate, and 3) that any program insofar as it gives primary emphasis (for either diagnosis or treatment) to "perception" (in whatever form) is not to be recommended.

The influence of gross motor exercises in the field of special education stems from their use with the mentally retarded. A pioneer in the training school movement, Edouard Seguin was much impressed with the Prussian drillmaster school of discipline that viewed a sound body as necessary to a sound mind (Talbot, 1964). No one has ever demonstrated that the motor clumsiness of the retarded was due to a lack of exercise and that motor dexterity would improve cognitive functioning. The leading proponent of this modality of therapy has been Kephart (1960, 1968). He sees development as a unidirectional and irreversible sequence from the motor through the perceptual to the conceptual. When cognitive deficits are noted in the older child, it is assumed that some type of muscular activity or sensorimotor experience was not fully integrated in infancy. The treatment program highlights the use of a walking beam to help the child internally map his body image; the laterality (internal) and directionality (external) of this body image are also emphasized. In the absence of any pressure, such motor coordination programs can act as a good recreational outlet in group athletics on a Saturday morning for the clumsy child who cannot keep up with his peers in gym class or who is never picked for neighborhood teams. They may even help to improve motor coordination. But they have no effect on learning.

Delacato (1959, 1963, 1966; cf. Doman, 1964) has proposed a theory of neurological organization that focuses on subcortical integration and the development of cortical dominance. The theoretical substrate for this approach is an extremely simplistic interpretation of Haeckel's "law" that ontogeny recapitulates phylogeny. (For the more complex truth contained in recapitulation, see de Beer, 1958). Thus the most primitive motor activities, suggestive of the mature patterns of lower species, are used to facilitate cognitive development. Proper cross-pattern creeping is practiced; parents are encouraged to passively impose a reverse asymmetrical tonic neck reflex posture (cf. Capute et al., 1978) on the sleeping child. Balance beams, trampolines, and eye exercises are also used in a comprehensive program to enhance the maturation of the central nervous system to its highest level, which is that of hemispheric dominance; music is prohibited since tonality is mediated by the nondominant hemisphere (cf. Masland and Cratty, 1972; Stainback, Stainback, and Hallahan, 1973). The therapeutic aspect of this theory is usually referred to as "patterning" and outcome studies do not appear to justify its use (Doman-Delacato Treatment of Neurologically Handicapped Children, 1968—a joint statement by seven professional organizations; Robbins and Glass, 1968; Zigler and Seitz, 1975). As S. A. Cohen (1969) concluded, one must teach children to read, not to crawl, or to cross pattern, or to draw triangles.

Delacato (1966) gave lucid expression to the key argument of all perceptual theories: reading is neither a conceptual nor an intellectual process; if it were, then children who could not read would also be unable to speak since it is the same language and the same brain. In both reading and speaking the conceptual content is the same; it is only the perceptual mode of presentation (visual as opposed to auditory) that is different; therefore, reading is a perceptual act. While children with reading problems do have expressive language, Delacato himself admits that reading disorders belong to one end of a spectrum of language disabilities; one of the most common findings in learning-disabled children is a history of early language delay, dysfluency, or dysarticulation. Second, the difference between spoken and written language is not merely the perceptual modality; there is also the concept of (as well as the specific type of) code. In Conan Doyle's "The Dancing Men," it must first be realized that the hieroglyphics are a code, and then the code must be broken. The resulting message (identical to the original "message") is English. Why does it take a Sherlock Holmes to unravel this? Why cannot any native speaker of English decipher the message? Perceptual problems aside, to claim that anyone who speaks English fluently can readily be taught to read English is similar to stating that anyone who can read English can easily master the art of cryptography. The child encountering beginning reading needs abstractive abilities of a high order and is not unlike the cryptanalyst trying to crack a cipher. Remember that when literacy was extremely rare, any piece of plain writing was a secret code to the mass of mankind (cf. Kahn, 1967).

Birch and Lefford (1963) suggested that children may have problems not within a specific perceptual mode but rather in crossing from one sensory modality to another. A number of studies documented the inferiority of learning-disabled children on a variety of tasks requiring intersensory integration using auditory, visual, haptic, and kinesthetic stimuli (Beery, 1967; Birch and Belmont, 1964; Whiton, Singer, and Cook, 1975). These studies failed, however, to control for verbal mediation: verbal or symbolic coding facilitates (if it is not absolutely necessary for) cross-modal sensory integration, and this is especially true when there is a temporal pattern involved (Blank and Bridger, 1966; Blank, Weider, and Bridger, 1968). Second, the factors of attention and memory were not appropriately controlled for (Vellutino, 1977). Last, a serious problem with cross-modal integration should itself severely affect the acquisition of spoken language (Rudel and Denckla, 1976).

Since the time of Hinshelwood, visual perception and its disorders have occupied an honored place in the field of learning disabilities. Yet visual-motor tests are not predictive of academic achievement (Haring and Ridgway, 1967), and visual sequential memory has only a moderate correlation with reading (Goldberg and Guthrie, 1972; Guthrie and Goldberg, 1972) and a good part of this relationship may depend on the memory and sequencing components of the task. As Clark (1970) concluded, practice on visual-perceptual items shows no transfer to word discrimination: the nearer the training is to the skill required, the more effective it will be.

The most elaborate approach to visual perception has been the Frostig Developmental Test of Visual Perception (DTVP), with its own remedial program. According to Frostig (1965a, b, 1972; Frostig and Maslow, 1969), visual perception consists of distinct subprocesses, each of which may be disturbed independent of the other. The five DTVP subtests are eye-hand coordination, figure-ground perception, perceptual constancy, position in space, and spatial relationships. Englehardt (1975), A. V. Olson (1968), and Sabatino, Abbott, and Becker (1974) have all questioned the content validity of the subtests; the DTVP measures only a single perceptual factor that is only weakly related to intelligence and not at all related to academic achievement (Colarusso, Martin, and Hartung, 1975; P. A. Smith and Marx, 1972). To try to use the subtests to obtain a profile analysis of areas of visual-perceptual strengths and weakness to aid in remediation would then appear to be an exercise in futility (cf. Mann, 1972). Working with Frostig materials improves performance on the DTVP; working with reading improves reading performance.

Auditory perception has received relatively less attention than visual perception, probably on the basis of the observation that children with reading problems speak and understand spoken language at a grossly normal level. Wepman (1962) reported that children with delayed auditory perception were slower in beginning to talk and in acquiring speech accuracy. A number of researchers have noted low scores on the Wepman Auditory Discrimination Test (R. Snyder and Pope, 1970; Wepman, 1958) in children with reading disorders (Capute et al., 1980; Clark, 1970). The test requires the examiner to read pairs of words that either are identical or differ in a single phoneme; the child must discriminate those pairs that are the same from those that are different. Obviously, in addition to auditory discrimination, successful performance on the test necessitates fair short-term memory, appropriate focusing of attention, and the conceptual understanding of same/different. Some severely hyperkinetic children will not be able to focus their attention adequately and actually seem to forget the first word by the time the second is spoken. As part of a general evaluation the instrument may be used, but careful clinical interpretation of the results is necessary.

In assessing auditory-perceptual abilities, most speech pathologists use subtests of the Illinois Test of Psycholinguistic Abilities (ITPA). This test is actually misnamed; reference to F. Smith and Miller (1966) or any other work on psycholinguistics will demonstrate little relationship to the subtest content of the ITPA. What the ITPA really taps are the auditory- and visual-perceptual processes presumed to underlie mature language function. The subtests include six at the representational level: an auditory and a visual reception (decoding), an auditory and a visual association, and a verbal and a manual expression (encoding); and four at the automatic level: a grammatic and a visual closure, and an auditory and a visual sequential memory (there are also two supplementary tests—auditory closure and sound blending) (see Lamb, 1969; Paraskevopoulos and Kirk, 1969). The test is unique in that it was specifically designed to aid in the diagnosis and treatment of learning disabilities. But research results have not been kind: ITPA subtests have been unable to distinguish learning-disabled from normal children (Hammill and Larsen, 1974a, b, 1978; Larsen, Rogers, and Sowell, 1976; cf. Lund, Foster, and McCall-Perez, 1978) and Carroll (1972) concluded that the resulting profile was not diagnostically superior to that of the WISC. Kirk and Kirk (1978) responded that the test had been misused and misinterpreted; although the published norms are for children between 2½ and 10 years of age, they suggested restricting its use to the 4- to 8-year range. Since many learning-disabled children are not identified until the second grade or later, this is a rather severe limitation. The real power of the ITPA was to be its recommendations for remediation based on a profile of auditory and visual strengths and weaknesses. Bateman (1969) matched and cross-matched a group of audile and visile learners (mean IQ 125) and found that the audile learners achieved more regardless of instructional mode, and a phonics approach (auditory synthesis) was superior regardless of the children's particular learning style. C. M. Smith (1971) repeated the study with a group of children whose mean IQ was 90 and again found no interaction between ITPA profiles, teaching methods, and levels of achievement (auditory superiority was not noted); these results question the validity of the ITPA and the concept of diagnostic-prescriptive teaching. It appears that children may not be bundles of isolated factors and processes, and teaching may require something more than the application of prepackaged remediation programs to the corresponding deficit patterns.

If sensation is an end-organ phenomenon and perception is a cortical phenomenon, then Ayres's sensory integration theory focuses on a hypothetical intermediate process that takes place in the brainstem. Ayres thus attempts to distinguish her approach from (and thereby avoid the current negative publicity attendant on) perceptual-motor approaches. She has developed a complex assessment battery, the Southern California Sensory Integration Tests (SCSIT) and an involved typology of learning-disabled children via factor analysis (Ayres, 1966, 1971, 1972a, b). Although much more elaborate than its predecessors, it seems to be perceptual-motor evaluation and training in new clothes. The perceptual roots of the SCSIT are readily revealed by the facts that, of the five tests that had been published separately before their inclusion in the battery, three have the word *perception* in the title, and the other two tests are: 1) "designed particularly for use with subjects. . . who have or are suspected of having perceptual difficulty," and 2) are designed "to assist in making diagnoses of perceptual motor dysfunction in young children" (see references in Buros, 1974). Although there does appear to be some positive correlation between tactile-perceptual functioning and reading ability (Finlayson and Reitan, 1976), this is probably mediated through general cortical function (IQ). Using the Southern California Battery, J. H. Meier (1971) could not distinguish learning-disabled children from controls. The published follow-up studies on sensory integration techniques are of short duration and utilize outcome measures like the Slosson (a brief version of the Stanford-Binet) and the Wide Range Achievement Test (WRAT, word recognition/decoding) in reading, perhaps the two least refined instruments available. J. D. Cohen (1976) complained that the field of learning disabilities is suffocating in such "correlation coefficients between fuzzies." Since it is probably possible to define a subgroup of learning-disabled children to correlate with just about anything, it is unlikely that the SCSIT will be the last example of "psychometric phrenology" (Mann, 1971b); "perception" exerts the attraction of an infinite variety.

Theories that are labeled sensory, sensorimotor, perceptual, perceptual-motor, auditory-perceptual, visual-motor, intersensory, or sensory-integrative have all been lumped together as "perceptual" for convenience; the common factor is their reliance for diagnosis and treatment upon hypothetical neurological precognitive processes as prerequisites to learning. In contrast, a cognitive approach to learning disorders focuses upon higher-order information processing. Thus poor readers have deficits in naming skills rather than visual perception (F. J. Morrison, Giordani, and Nagy, 1977); they have difficulty in integrating and retrieving verbal equivalents (Vellutino, Steger, and Kandel, 1972). Reading-disabled children neither code (label) nor synthesize (chunk) information as readily as normal children do (Vellutino, 1977); they differ in their responses to visual and tactile stimuli only on measures involving a verbal component (Vellutino, Bentley, and Phillips, 1978). Even the classic orientation errors such as *b* for *d* and *was* for *saw* are a function of verbal identification rather than optical distortion (Vellutino et al., 1975).

PERCEPTUAL CONCLUSIONS

1. It is doubtful whether a specific volume of perceptual experience is necessary before conceptualization can occur (Mac-Keith, 1977); if such a quantity exists, the qualitative aspects of the required experience are almost totally unknown. Several valid hypotheses have been posed for normal cognitive development; the range of successful spontaneous accommodations available to children with various neurological impairments is not known.

2. Processes subsumed under the heading "perceptual" are not passive building blocks for higher functions; they are themselves the products of abstraction and hypothesis construction (cf. Neisser, 1967).

3. Training perception (and other neurological substrates of learning) may (or may not) improve perception, but it has little to no effect on learning (Balow, 1971; Hammill, 1972). The converse is *not* true: reading delays may be raised to normal levels through reading instruction despite the persistance of significant visual-perceptual motor disorders (M. E. Robinson and Schwartz, 1973).

4. Although perceptual training is ineffective in learning disabilities, the screening for perceptual disorders uncovers phenomena that have some correlation to learning problems (Sapir and Wilson, 1978). These perceptual deficits should be considered cognitive soft signs and should receive the same cautious interpretation within the context of the total clinical picture that neurological soft signs require.

5. The categorization of specific learning disability (SLD) children by perceptual types does not appear to affect outcome. Although educationally it seems to be a safe assumption that it is helpful for a teacher to know whether a child is an audile or a visile learner, a good teacher will probably recognize this before any formal evaluation, it is undecided whether teaching to strengths or weaknesses is optimal, and good teaching automatically includes whatever perceptual training is necessary.

6. The diagnosis of a "perceptual deficit" is little more than a restatement of the fact that a child is having learning difficul-

ties and tells nothing about the nature or origin of the problem (Schain, 1973).

7. Most psychological tests of perception or related pseudoneurological processes have questionable construct validity (Larsen, 1976) and poor statistical reliability (Sabatino, 1979)—so much so that their use for individual diagnosis or educational programming is inappropriate.

8. As an etiology or a treatment modality for learning disorders, perception does not exist, and what does not exist cannot be trained (Mann, 1971a). There has been a "serious overinvestment in the leaky hypostatizations of perception" from the point of view of education (Mann, 1972).

LEARNING DISABILITY AND LANGUAGE

The idea that learning disabilities reflect underlying disorders of linguistic competence is gaining increasing acceptance. Dyslexia and other types of learning disability are best understood when placed on a spectrum of developmental disorders of language (Ingram, 1960a, b, 1975) or a language continuum (D. J. Johnson, 1968). Much of the confusing and contradictory research on perceptual problems in learning disability is best explained by a language hypothesis in which perceptual impairments actually represent a more fundamental involvement of conceptual and symbolic processes. Thus perceptual disturbances are secondary phenomena; the language disorder that is at the root of learning disabilities inhibits verbalization from stabilizing perception (A. L. Benton, 1962, 1968; de Hirsch, 1973; Luria, 1961; Luria and Yudovich, 1971).

A delay in early language milestones is common in learning-disabled children (Capute et al., 1980; Denhoff, 1973b; Mason, 1967; Rutter, 1972; Tarnopol, 1969b), and those dyslexic children who were late in talking actually appear to have a worse prognosis. Such early language delay may be found to occur even more frequently when language milestones are elicited sequentially using a carefully graded scale (Capute and Accardo, 1978). Apart from delay, deviance or an abnormal acquisition sequence may be even more significant. Since language is probably the best predictor of future achievement, it is unfortunate that infant development tests emphasize sensorimotor skills rather than linguistic milestones. There is no acceptable predictor of future learning disabilities in children, but if one is ever developed (in the face of serious theoretical prohibitions; see section on early screening), it will be heavily weighted with early language development.

It is interesting that premature infants with various risk factors "caught up" in perceptual and cognitive development by 2 years of age, but that their language skills were noticeably different (Zarin-Ackerman, Lewis, and Driscoll, 1977). Apart from early language delays, older learning-disabled and dyslexic children demonstrate subtle but significant deficiencies in their ability to handle syntactic information (Vogel, 1975) as well as in their expressive language, which tends to be less fluent, less complex, and less grammatically correct (M. A. Fry, Johnson, and Muehl, 1970).

The presentation of the early language delay may be quite deceptive. One child presented at 3 years of age with no speech, severe mental retardation, and unmanageable behavior; an intensive therapeutic program boosted her IQ into the genius range after controlling the behavior. When reexamined at 9 years of age, the child demonstrated normal intelligence, a significant learning disability, verbal dysfluency, and an obvious mild right hemiplegia. There was a fairly clear history of a cerebral insult late in the first year of life, and apparently the transfer of language dominance to the right hemisphere was incomplete or limited.

Since expressive language (vocalization) is usually considered to be distinct from receptive language (comprehension), dysarticulation is related to oral motor apraxia rather than to true linguistic competence. Reality, however, does not allow such a clear separation of these two aspects of language: in addition to an early history of delayed language milestones, many learning-disabled children also present with articulation problems (Capute et al., 1980; Hart et al., 1974; L. I. Lawson, 1965; Rutter, 1972; Templin, 1966). A survey of 11-year-old school children demonstrated that a persisting articulation disorder was strongly associated with poor attainment in all scholastic areas (Calnan and Richardson, 1977). Even a dysarticulation that undergoes spontaneous remission in the preschool years can be a developmental marker of high risk for a later learning disability. When seen at school age, the child with a history of dysarticulation but whose speech is now normal may express his fundamental language disability as a learning disorder rather than as a speech problem. Thus, in a 5-year follow-up of children originally seen between 3 and 8 years of age for speech or language delay, less than 10% were performing at grade level (Gofman and Allmond, 1971b). The underlying disability remains the same, the mode of expression changes with age and circumstances.

EARLY DETECTION

At first the Infant,
Mewling, and puking in the Nurses armes:
Then, the whining Schoole-boy with his Satchell
And shining morning face, creeping like snaile
Unwilling to schoole.

Shakespeare,
As You Like It

INFANCY

Knobloch and Pasamanick (1959) considered sucking difficulties
and abnormalities of tone in the first month of life to be suggestive of later minimal brain dysfunction (MBD). Laufer and Denhoff (1957) described hyperactive children as exhibiting hypertonicity, colic, and sleep disturbances in infancy; Denhoff (1973a)
characterized such children as having been difficult-to-manage
babies, overreactive to stimuli like light or noise. In a study of
twin pairs, Matheny, Dolan, and Wilson (1976) identified the following behavioral antecedents of learning disability in infancy:
sleep disturbances, feeding problems, intense temper, increased
activity level, and distractibility.

Children who will later develop MBD/specific learning disability (SLD) are frequently suspected of more severe neurological
disturbances in infancy. Of a group of children who were diagnosed as spastic cerebral palsy or developmental delay under 1
year of age and were considered normal by 3 years of age, approximately one-third later turned out to have MBD (Denhoff, 1973b).
Similarly, one-third of children with neurological dysfunction in
the newborn period, when followed to 9 years of age, were backward in school performance, with poor language development and
impaired fine motor control (Francis-Williams, 1976). Both major
and minor neurological symptoms at birth and 1 year are associated with academic problems at 7 years of age (Denhoff, Hainsworth, and Hainsworth, 1972). Even transient (disappearing by 8
days of age) neonatal signs, such as jitteriness, shivering, restlessness, frog posturing, and limpness, have been related to some
limitation of intellectual performance at school age (Mednick,
1977).

Prechtl (1960, 1963) described three neurobehavioral syndromes identifiable in the newborn period: apathy, hemisyn-
drome, and hyperexcitability. This last syndrome consisted of

infants with vigorous suck, hypertonicity, excessive crying, sudden changes of state, exaggerated reflexes with low thresholds (especially the Moro reflex), and a limb tremor (high amplitude 4–6/second) during spontaneous activity. Many of these hyperexcitable infants later developed the choreiform syndrome; if the hyperexcitable syndrome had been present in a child with other risk factors, as many as three-quarters exhibited the choreiform syndrome in later childhood (Prechtl, 1961, 1965). In the New York Longitudinal Study, Thomas and Chess (1977) used nine behavioral categories—activity level, rhythmicity (regularity), approach/withdrawal, adaptability, threshold of responsiveness, intensity of reaction, quality of mood, distractibility, and attention span/persistence—to characterize temperament in infancy; 40% of babies fit an easy child temperament, with 10% in the difficult child, 15% in the slow-to-warm-up child, and 35% in mixed categories. Whereas the difficult child constellation (high intensity, negative moods, and arrhythmicity) signaled a high incidence of behavioral manifestations in mentally retarded children, school problems demonstrated a stronger association with the slow-to-warm-up pattern (nonadaptable, withdrawn).

These neurobehavioral syndromes should never be considered as diagnostic in infancy. The use of methylphenidate in infancy, recommended by some (cf. Denhoff, 1973a; Nichamin, 1972), should never be necessary. Rather these clinical findings can be used by the pediatrician to counsel the parents of infants with minimal neurological dysfunction. Because these babies are easily startled, a mother often has the impression of frightening her baby; she thinks that she is mishandling the infant (Prechtl, 1961). Many such children seem to find the normal amount of mothering inadequate (Laufer and Denhoff, 1957). Maternal tension increases with the degree of neurological damage (Knobloch and Pasamanick, 1966). In the anticipatory guidance that is the routine function of the pediatrician, it must be kept in mind that neurologically abnormal babies do not make adequate partners in the child-maternal interaction. Indeed, mothers of babies who are grossly abnormal seem to adjust better than mothers whose infants are only minimally involved, since the latter mothers often do not realize that the baby is contributing to the problem (Prechtl, 1963). These mothers will be comforted and better able to handle such infants when they are helped to realize that the problem is manageable and not their fault. The most damaging error committed by many professionals involved with mothers and infants is to ignore the signs of neurological dysfunction in the infant and to assume that all the blame is to be placed on inadequate mothering. Parents of handicapped children have enough problems with feelings of guilt without having them exaggerated by the very professionals whose role it is to help.

EARLY SCREENING

What can only be described as an obsession with early diagnosis has led to a proliferation of early (mostly at the kindergarten level) screening instruments. Table 7 compares the component elements of several such batteries; their reliance on perceptual-motor items is obvious. De Hirsch et al. (1966) started with 37 tests in kindergarten; they found that 19 related significantly to overall reading performance at the end of second grade and from these selected a diagnostic index of 10 tests and a screening index of five tests. The screening index predicts reading failure with a true positive rate of 75%; its false positive rate is approximately 25% (Jansky and de Hirsch, 1972). A. A. Silver et al. (1976) developed SEARCH as a 20-minute battery to be administered at the end of kindergarten or the beginning of first grade; children with low scores have a 90% incidence of definite neurological dysfunction. The Abbreviated Screening Battery (Satz and Friel, 1978), given at the beginning of kindergarten, will detect 90% of those identified as severely learning disabled at the end of second grade while only misclassifying 18% of normal children. Ozer's (1968) 15-minute neurological evaluation is included here rather than in the discussion of soft signs because of its learning components. Denhoff et al. (1968) reported on their experience with the Meeting Street School Screening Test (MSSST); when 4 or more out of the total 36 tests were failed, approximately half of these children experienced significant academic failure; for this same cutoff the false positive rate was approximately 50% and the false negative rate was 5%. Dubowitz, Leibowitz, and Goldberg (1977) devised a 10-minute screening assessment to correlate with the Wechsler Preschool and Primary Scale of Intelligence (WPPSI); it includes constructing block figures, copying the Gesell drawings, counting fingers, grouping cubes, and digit span. Reimer et al. (1975) presented a practical scoring technique for name printing for 5½- to

Table 7. Screening instruments

Gesell readiness	Predictive index
1. Write name	1. Pencil use
2. Write numbers	2. Bender Gestalt (5)
3. Copy geometric forms	3. Wepman Auditory
4. Incomplete man	Discrimination (20)
5. R-L discrimination	4. Number of words in telling
6. Matching/reproducing	a story
designs	5. Categories
7. Name animals (1 minute)	6. Horst reversals
	7. Gates word matching
	8. Word recognition I
	9. Word recognition II
	10. Word reproduction

Screening index	Preschool Readiness Experimental Screening Scale (PRESS)
1. Letter naming	1. Knowledge of colors
2. Picture naming	2. Digit span
3. Binet sentence memory	3. General information
4. Gates word matching	4. Drawing coordination
5. Bender-Gestalt	

6½-year-old children in the last 10 weeks of kindergarten. Cowgill, Friedland, and Shapiro (1973) had kindergarten teachers rate children on maturity, attention span, motor control, social and emotional adjustment, popularity, and speech and language; Haring and Ridgway (1967) used kindergarten teachers' observations in 11 different areas. Both of these studies suggest that despite wide individual variations, the broad behavioral samplings enabled a fairly accurate identification of future underachievers. Other scales have been proposed by Novack, Bonaventura, and Merenda (1973) and Sapir and Wilson (1967). Recently N. L. Kaufman and Kaufman (1974) and A. S. Kaufman and Kaufman (1977a, b) noted that the General Cognitive Index (GCI) from the McCarthy Scales of Children's Abilities (McCarthy, 1972) demonstrates a 15- to 20-point discrepancy from the IQ in MBD underachievers, and they recommend its use as a screening instrument. As a formal psychometric instrument for children between 2½ and 8½ years

Table 7– *continued*

SEARCH	Abbreviated screening battery
Visual	*Factor I (sensorimotor-perceptual)*
1. Discrimination	1. Finger localization
2. Recall	2. Recognition-discrimination
3. Visual motor	
Auditory	*Factor II (verbal-conceptual)*
4. Discrimination	3. Beery Developmental Test of
5. Rote sequencing	Visual Motor Integration
	4. PPVT
Intermodal	5. Dichotic listening
6. Spoken	
7. Written	*Factor III (verbal-cultural)*
	6. Wepman Auditory Discrimination
Body image (neurological	7. Alphabet recitation
development)	8. SES
8. Directionality	
9. Finger localization	
10. Pencil grasp	

Neurological evaluation of school-age children	
Motor	*Nonmotor*
1. Stand on one foot	9. R-L discrimination
2. Heel-to-toe gait	10. Articulation
3. Foot tapping	11. Face-hand test
4. Hop in place	12. Auditory distractibility
5. Complex synergistic	13. Figure-ground discrimination
movement	*Unspecified*
6. Finger-to-nose test	14. Position sense
7. Fine finger movements	15. OKN
8. Rapid lip/tongue	16. Two-point discrimination
movements	17. Haptic reproduction

Data from Ames (1968b), de Hirsch et al. (1966), Jansky and de Hirsch (1972), W. B. Rogers and Rogers (1972), A. A. Silver et al. (1976), Satz and Friel (1978), Yahraes and Prestwich (1976), Ozer (1968), and Kohen-Raz (1977).

of age, the McCarthy is in a different category from the above screening instruments, and the preliminary results with GCI warrant further investigation.

The dogma that early intervention resulting from early screening and diagnosis will eventuate in an improved prognosis for the learning-disabled child is an article of faith open to attack on several grounds. First, there is absolutely no evidence to support this hypothetical association (cf. Alberman, 1973). Second, the very proliferation of screening tests suggests an inverse Gresham's law: if any of these instruments were really effective predictors, they would drive the others from the marketplace. Since several of these batteries are fairly recent, perhaps one of them will become *the* screening instrument. A conservative skepticism might alternatively suggest that the preliminary statistics obtained with these experimental batteries (partially a result of the initial enthusiasm attaching to all such projects) are now at their best and will ultimately decline if and when these instruments achieve more widespread use. This eventuality is itself unlikely since the first response of many clinicians to such batteries is to pick and choose those items that suit their own theoretical bias on the nature of learning disabilities. (Indeed, taking the end of second grade reading level as the outcome measure must raise some doubt as to validity; see Appendix B.) Third, the very possibility of screening must be seriously questioned. The kindergarten age span covers a transitional period with rapid changes in many areas (in Gesell's terminology, an age of disequilibrium; see Ames, 1968a); this very acceleration of developmental trends makes point estimations of functional levels exceedingly hazardous. This developmental phenomenon helps to explain the range of false positive rates of at least 10% to 20%; it remains a moral issue for society whether such a rate is acceptable for the purposes of labeling and the institution of compensatory programs. Fourth, while operational definitions may help avoid some of the terminological confusion, it remains that early screening and the related intervention programs are aimed at preventing or ameliorating disorders: 1) whose very existence has been questioned, 2) whose diagnosis and definition in the target older child are the subject of much disagreement, and 3) whose remediation (as to both type and efficacy) is debated. Commitment to any kind of screening program will require educators to thoroughly revise a number of their basic assumptions with regard to child development if they are to escape a catch-22 logic. Thus, Satz and Friel (1978) noted that without any formal assessment kindergarten teachers could predict approximately 80% of future learning-disabled children (the same order of magnitude for true positives as any screening battery), but for official placement purposes, these same teachers reported only a quarter of such children out of a fear of mislabeling. In other words, a large part of the learning-disabled population can be identified early without the use of refined screening devices; what prevents this from actually happening is a deep-rooted philosophical ambivalence that will not be easily eradicated by some brief "objective" screening procedure.

From a pediatric perspective much of this discussion of screening seems to betray a fundamental ignorance of the complexities of development. The value of a developmental assessment is inversely proportional to the time invested; therefore, the pediatrician never "screens" development. Rather, he assesses it, and not at one critical age but repeatedly at multiple well-child checkups. He accumulates a knowledge of relevant perinatal and familial factors in addition to developmental patterns throughout infancy and early childhood. He looks at school readiness skills more from a qualitative aspect, frequently utilizing techniques of interpretation developed by Haeussermann (1958; Jedrysek et al., 1972) to elicit minor central nervous system involvement in cerebral palsied children. The outcome of the pediatric assessment is not a label leading to class placement in an early intervention program of unproved merit but a clinical diagnosis of at risk, a recommendation for a trial of school (Ozer, 1968), and a careful follow-up of school attitudes and academic progress. When a learning disability is finally diagnosed by an *actual* failure in achievement, then the pediatrician supports whatever special help appears appropriate.

PEDIATRIC NEURO-DEVELOPMENTAL EVALUATION

Some circumstantial evidence is very strong, as when you find a trout in the milk.

Thoreau,
Journal

While problems with rhyming (Gibson and Levin, 1975), difficulties in naming colors (Rutter, 1969), and the persistence of reversals ("the deadly sin of reversals"—Kinsbourne, 1973b) have some attraction as developmental markers, there is no single pathognomonic sign to make a diagnosis of specific learning disability (SLD). This qualification holds true for medicine, psychology, and education and necessitates an interdisciplinary evaluation. A comprehensive pediatric assessment needs to focus on: 1) a detailed developmental history, 2) an expanded neurological examination, 3) a careful physical examination to detect minor physical anomalies, 4) a battery of drawing tests, and 5) a brief psychoeducational evaluation. The resulting neurodevelopmental profile can then be integrated with the findings of the other members of the multidisciplinary team.

EXPANDED NEUROLOGICAL EXAMINATION

The most controversial and confused area in the pediatrics of learning disabilities concerns interpretation of the soft neurological signs of the expanded neurological examination. For some, "soft signs" are evaluated by the soft-headed pediatrician, while "hard signs" are noted by the hard-headed neurologist. In a more serious vein, however, the traditional or classical neurological signs (i.e., hard signs) have a unitary and localizing significance; the normal response does not change and, in combination with other hard signs, an abnormal response indicates a specific locus of neuropathology. The nontraditional or paraclassical soft signs, on the other hand, are developmental; that is, the "correct" response changes with age. Failure to consider this maturational factor has led soft signs to be classed as minor, equivocal, intermittent, and unreliable. Certainly, having ascertained their presence, no single interpretation is compulsory; they may reflect either damage or delay in the central nervous system. As Denhoff et al. (1968) suggested, they measure function rather than directly assess pathology, and in many cases they are actually tapping higher cortical processes (cf. Erickson, 1977; Gofman and Allmond, 1971b).

Another reason for the "softness" of these signs of minor neurological dysfunction is the lack of a standardized battery and accepted methods for eliciting individual signs. Touwen and Prechtl's (1970; revised edition Touwen, 1979) manual cannot be said to have achieved very widespread use—except piecemeal and with variations, which vitiates its contribution. Despite variability on serial examinations (McMahon and Greenberg, 1977), soft signs can demonstrate a high interexaminer reliability (Werry et al., 1972) and consistency in individual patients (Kennard, 1960). All the studies for and against soft signs utilize a different selection of items; every paper presents innovations in scoring, and many researchers try to devise briefer assessments focusing on *the* soft sign that will distinguish the deviant child. Criticizing such work is easy; comparing the results is difficult; complete lack of agreement with their goals is necessary.

Touwen and Sporrel (1979) pointed out that soft signs diagnose the presence of minor neurological dysfunction (MND); the problem is the relationship between MND and neurobehavioral syndromes, such as minimal brain dysfunction (MBD), SLD, and dyslexia. Soft signs might best be considered neurodevelopmental markers (cf. Rutter, 1977) and compared to the four-finger palmar flexion crease in Down syndrome. A simian crease occurs in 50% of trisomy 21 patients and in approximately 10% of normal subjects. Since normals vastly outnumber patients with Down syndrome, if one used the crease as a screening test for either Down syndrome or mental retardation, one's yield would be fairly poor. (With 14 Down syndrome patients in a population of 10,000 there would be 7 true positives, 8,987 true negatives, 7 false negatives, and 999 false positives.) In combination with a dozen other anomalies, the simian crease is fairly diagnostic of Down syndrome, but the definitive test is an abnormal karyotype. However, both before and after the chromosomal examination, the patient will be examined and the associated anomalies noted. Similarly, soft signs are not particularly diagnostic; although they may contribute to the identification of distinct neurobehavioral syndromes (Touwen, 1979), they should never be used to screen for learning or behavioral disorders—the number of false positives and false negatives is too great.

Between one-third (Hart et al., 1974; Kenny and Clemmens, 1972; Kenny et al., 1972) and one-half (Wolcott, 1972) of children with learning problems demonstrate significant soft neurological signs. Whether as indices of maturational delay or mild brain damage, soft signs might contribute to identifying which of those children with developmental clumsiness (developmental apraxia, congenital maladroitness, the clumsy child syndrome) are at greater risk for learning problems (cf. Gubbay et al., 1965; Illingworth, 1963; Reuben and Bakwin, 1968). There does not appear to be any relationship between soft signs and electroencephalographic (EEG) abnormalities (Hart et al., 1974; Kennard, 1960), nor is there any strong correlation with reading disability (Kennard, 1960). Using a battery of 10 to 12 soft signs, Satterfield et al. (1973; Satterfield, Lesser, Saul, and Cantwell, 1973) demonstrated a scale of increasing responsiveness to medication for hyperactivity as one moved from group one to group four: 1) normal EEG and normal neurological examination, 2) normal EEG and abnormal neurological examination, 3) abnormal EEG and normal neurological examination, 4) abnormal EEG and abnormal neurological examination.

The most common types of soft signs evaluated involve synkinesias, or associated movements. These superfluous movements are unnecessary to the action they accompany; they are usually contralateral and symmetric to that part voluntarily in action (Connolly and Stratton, 1968). Both contralateral and ipsilateral synkinesias show a marked decline after 9 years of age (H. J. Cohen et al., 1967; Twitchell et al., 1966); voluntary suppression of mirror movements develops between 5 and 6½ years of age (Kohen-Raz, 1977). The overshooting of movements into other muscle groups (Lucas et al., 1965) is even more obvious in frank brain damage syndromes, such as cerebral palsy; impairment of the later-developing inhibitory mechanisms releases the more primitive excitatory mechanisms responsible for mirror movements. (In hemiplegia the overflow is greater to the involved side.) With general cognitive delay, a failure of internalized representation of movements probably contributes to the synkinesia; the underlying mechanism for the mirroring seen in the Klippel-Feil anomolad (brevicollis, torticollis, webbed neck, and Sprengel's deformity) is unclear, but it is probably distinct from the above and related to more peripheral (orthopedic) factors. H. J. Cohen et al. (1967) have demonstrated that associated movements are inde-

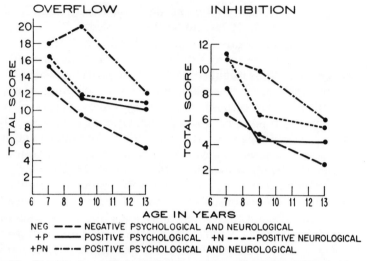

OVERFLOW

INHIBITION

AGE IN YEARS

NEG ━ ━ ━ NEGATIVE PSYCHOLOGICAL AND NEUROLOGICAL
+P ━━━━ POSITIVE PSYCHOLOGICAL   +N ━ ━ ━ ━ POSITIVE NEUROLOGICAL
+PN ━·━·━ POSITIVE PSYCHOLOGICAL AND NEUROLOGICAL

Figure 12.   Decrease in overflow movements with age. Chronological age, mental age, and the presence of organic brain damage all independently affect the presence and degree of overflow movements. The more involved children demonstrate scores similar to younger normal children. The right half of the figure (inhibition) shows a lowering of quantitated overflow for all groups when the subjects were instructed to voluntarily inhibit the overflow. (From H. J. Cohen et al., Developmental changes in overflow in normal and aberrantly functioning children, *Journal of Pediatrics 71*, pp. 39–47, © 1967, with permission.)

pendently affected by age, intelligence, and brain damage (Figure 12). Synkinesias are also influenced by the complexity of the movement, the intensity, the order of presentation, the familiarity of the task, and lateralization, with the nondominant side exhibiting more overflow (Touwen, 1979).

That the expanded neurological examination is "almost irrelevant" (P. H. Wender, 1971) or produces so little meaningful information as to be useless (Kenny and Clemmens, 1972; Kenny et al., 1972) are criticisms that apply only when soft signs are employed in a "witch hunt for the abnormal neuron" (Gofman and Allmond, 1971b). Such neurological signs by themselves cannot lead to a diagnosis; although they can statistically discriminate MBD children from matched controls (Denckla and Rudel, 1978; Erickson, 1977; Peters et al., 1974; Peters, Romine, and Dykman, 1975; Table 8), these are group results and of little help in the evaluation of individual children unless carefully integrated with other relevant medical and nonmedical findings.

Table 8. Neurological examination for minimal brain dysfunction

1. Passive head rotation— arms drop or spread	1. Strabismus
2. Copy finger movements	2. Nystagmus
3. Hop on one foot (8 feet)	3. FFM
4. Skip	4. RAM
5. FFM	5. Fingers between
6. RAM	6. Tactile identification
7. Index finger/thumb tapping	7. Graphesthesia
8. Associated movements in above	8. Outstretched arms
9. R-L confusion	9. Heel-to-toe gait
10. Head movement with EOM	10. Hop on one foot
11. Dysfluent speech	11. Skip
12. Dysgraphia	

The first column, from Peters et al. (1974), and the second column, from Erickson (1977), list soft neurological signs that discriminate between control and subject populations.

CHOREIFORM MOVEMENTS

When the upper extremities are flexed at the shoulders and extended at the elbows so that the outstretched arms are parallel to one another and to the floor, the most common minor neurological sign observed is a posture of overpronation with some wrist flexion, finger extension, and overabduction of the fourth and fifth fingers to produce the avoiding response, also described as spooning, bayonet, or dinner fork posture (Twitchell et al., 1966). Drifting should also be noted; according to Schilder's test (the same posture with the eyes closed), the dominant arm will be held somewhat higher than the nondominant one. Peripheral jerking in the fingers and hands are characterized as choreiform movements. Evaluating hyperactive children between 9 and 12 years of age, Prechtl and Stemmer (1962) noticed a high incidence of muscle artifacts on EEG; a closer reexamination of their patients revealed choreiform twitching (sudden, jerky, slight, of short duration) of the extremities distally and (more prominent) of the tongue, face, and neck proximally. Approximately two-thirds of these children had had obstetrical or postnatal problems and many fit the newborn classification of hyperexcitability syndrome. Many demonstrated brisk deep tendon reflexes and knee clonus, but their overall motor coordination could be quite good, with a paucity of other minor neurological signs; they were also noted to be accident prone (Prechtl, 1962).

Since Prechtl's first description of this choreiform syndrome, its significance has been questioned. Rutter, Graham, and Birch (1966) found the choreiform movements to be unreliable and very variable in a single child; although the chorea decreased with age and increasing intelligence level, when these factors were controlled, there was no significant relationship to reading disorders, psychiatric disturbances, neurological abnormalities, or perinatal complications. On the other hand, Wolff and Hurwitz (1966) reported choreiform movements to occur with significantly greater frequency in learning disabilities, emotional disorders, and juvenile delinquency. Even within a large population of normal children, the presence of the choreiform syndrome related to scholastic achievement and behavioral difficulties (Wolff and Hurwitz, 1973). When trying to interpret these data, it must be remembered that: 1) 12% of all children (both American and Japanese) exhibit choreiform movements (Wolff and Hurwitz, 1966), but 2) the choreiform syndrome accounts for a very small proportion of MBD children.

MOTOR IMPERSISTENCE

Many children with minor neurological dysfunction exhibit "motor unrest" (Boshes and Myklebust, 1964), an inability to sustain voluntary motor acts that is suggestive of bilateral or diffuse cerebral involvement (Garfield, 1964). A number of simple tasks (e.g., keeping eyelids closed, mouth open, tongue protruded, or gaze fixed laterally) need only to be observed for 20 seconds during the routine pediatric examination in order to elicit this sign. The child's initial success proves that he understands what is expected, so it does not appear to reflect a problem with cognition or perception.

GAIT

Children should be able to hop on either foot by 5 years of age, to stand on one leg by 6 years of age, to skip by 7 years of age, and to tandem walk (walk a straight line with alternate heels and toes touching) by 9 years of age (Page-El and Grossman, 1973; Vuckovich, 1968). Whereas the classical neurological examination focuses on gait disturbances as reflective of long tract (pyramidal) or cerebellar disturbances, the expanded neurological examination interprets minor deviations or clumsiness as indicative of higher-level (cortical) dysfunction. Thus, on heel and toe gaits vertical synkinesias are considered significant: on his heels, the child flexes his elbows and hyperextends his wrists, while on his toes the child tends to extend his elbows and palmar flex his wrists (Hart et al., 1974; McMahon and Greenberg, 1977).

FOG TEST

The Fog test (Fog and Fog, 1963) is another gait test to elicit vertical synkinesia. There are two versions of this foot-to-hands test: the direct form, in which the patient walks on the outsides (lateral or external soles) of his feet (inverted), and the indirect form, in which the patient walks on the insides (medial or inner) soles of his feet (everted). The patient is instructed to try to keep his arms down by his sides. The posturing of the upper extremities induced by these maneuvers (Figure 13) have been described as infantile (Twitchell et al., 1966) and they also strongly resemble ones seen in cerebral palsied patients. These associated movements should disappear between 10 and 13 years of age, but the test may be used qualitatively in younger children. The two distinct advantages to this particular gait test are that it correlates less well with other soft signs (Connolly and Stratton, 1968) and it is one of the last signs to disappear in adolescence.

FINE FINGER MOVEMENTS (FFM)

By 38 months of age most children have the motor ability to oppose the thumb to each of the other four fingers on the same hand in succession (Kuhlman, 1939); between 3 and 8 years of age this ability becomes more refined (Lefford, Birch, and Green, 1974), but mirror movements in the opposite hand do not disappear until 10 years of age (Grant, Boelsche, and Zin, 1973; Touwen and Prechtl, 1970). The difficulty that younger children have with this task seems to result from their not flexing the fingers enough; Twitchell et al. (1966) have interpreted this as an exaggeration of the avoiding response. The test may be repeated, with the child instructed to inhibit overflow to the opposite hand. Variations on

A

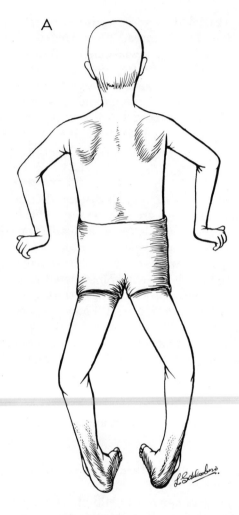

Figure 13A.   Fog test, direct form.

this item include tapping the thumb and index finger together as
rapidly as possible and tapping rhythmic patterns in imitation
(Close, 1973; Denckla, 1973; Hurwitz et al., 1972). Differential
dexterity in these tasks may be used as an indication of hand dominance (Adams et al., 1974).

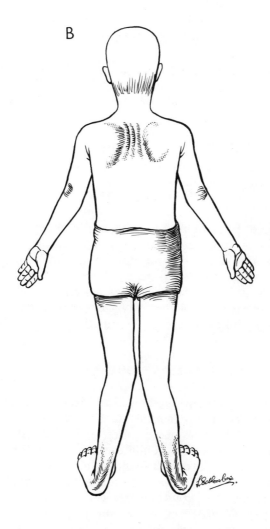

B

Figure 13B.   Fog test, indirect form.

DIADOCHOKINESIS

By 7 to 8 years of age the child is able to smoothly and rapidly pro-
nate/supinate his forearms while lightly slapping the dorsal and
plantar surfaces of his hands against his knees (Grant et al., 1973;
Touwen, 1979). Clumsiness on these rapid alternating movements
(RAM) is referred to as dysdiadochokinesis; when done with one
hand at a time, overflow may be looked for.

FACE-HAND TEST

Double simultaneous stimuli are applied to the face and hand while the child's eyes are closed; the stimulus to the hand is the one most frequently extinguished (not noticed). The test is not useful under 6 years of age, but by 7 years of age normal children will rarely make more than 1 error out of 10 trials (Fink and Bender, 1953; Kraft, 1968; Page-El and Grossman, 1973).

FINGER-TO-NOSE TEST

The child places the tip of his index finger alternately on the tip of his nose and the tip of the examiner's index finger, which is at arm's length from the child and may be moving or stationary. Dysmetria (overshooting) or tremor on this test in the classical neurological examination is considered a sign of cerebellar dysfunction, but in the expanded neurological examination it is interpreted as a sign of minor cortical dysfunction.

MISCELLANEOUS SIGNS

Mildly brisk or slightly asymmetrical deep tendon reflexes (DTRs) may reflect minor neurological involvement. Irregular oscillations or mild nystagmoid jerks on lateral gaze may be noted; the child may exhibit a unilateral winking deficit (Wikler, Dixon, and Parker, 1970) or a difficulty in elevating his eyebrows (Twitchell et al., 1966). By 9 years of age the child should be able to puff out his cheeks alternately and uniformly and whistle (Page-El and Grossman, 1973). When testing for graphesthesia (writing numbers with pressure on the palms), the child should be oriented correctly (Adams et al., 1974; Close, 1973). Some finger-spreading tests (e.g., "Vulcan salute") are not very helpful since more than half of 15-year-olds still demonstrate associated movements (Connolly and Stratton, 1968). Fog and Fog (1963) also used the pinching of bulldog clips as a stress to elicit mirror movements. Some items from Bergès and Lézine's (1965) scales for the imitation of gestures are depicted in Figure 14. Christensen (1975) has provided a detailed manual for Luria's neuropsychological investigation.

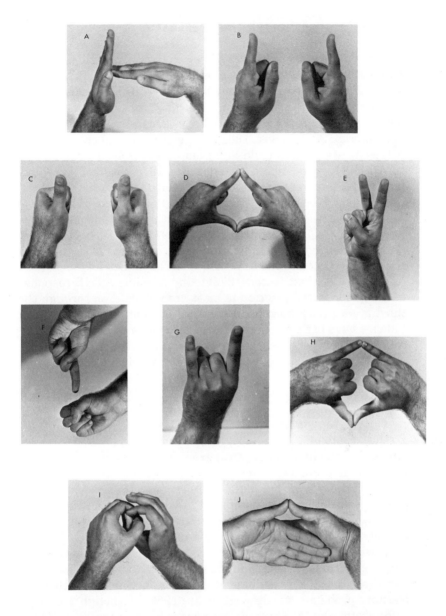

Figure 14.   Imitation of gestures. Selected items from Bergès and Lézine (1965) to assess perception and praxis in young children. A is item 5 from Imitation of Simple Gestures: Hand Movements; B through J are items 1, 2, 3, 5, 6, 8, 10, 11, and 12 from Imitation of Complex Gestures: Hand and Finger Movements. By 4 years of age, 75% of normal children will be able to imitate B, C, D; by 5 years, A, F, I; by 6 years, E; by 7 years, G. H.

PRIMITIVE REFLEXES

In cerebral palsy, primitive reflexes persist well beyond infancy; if minimal brain dysfunction is a mild form of cerebral palsy, some traces of primitive reflexes may be found (cf. Capute et al., 1978). Kennard (1960) described the "whirling" phenomenon—as the head turns, the upper half of the body turns with it on the body's long axis (cf. A. A. Silver, 1961). Hyperextension of the trunk and extremities when the child is placed in the prone extension posture (PEP) has been noted (Ottenbacher, 1978). Both of these findings may be expressions of a residual tonic labyrinthine reflex or reflections of vestibular dysfunction. Persistence of primitive reflexes has been noted as characteristic of certain subgroups of learning-disabled children (Ayres, 1971, 1972a, b). Critchley (1970) attributed lateral deviation of the outstretched arms when the head is turned to the influence of the asymmetrical tonic neck reflex (ATNR); Parmenter (1975) found a visible ATNR response in the quadrupedal position in most normal children through the third grade. With current methods of evaluation, such postural reflexes have little to contribute to the evaluation of the individual child; their persistence is, however, correlated in large groups with a higher occurrence of behavior problems (Finocchiaro, 1974).

MINOR PHYSICAL ANOMALIES

Gross abnormalities on physical examination are rare in learning-disabled children. While head circumferences more than 2 standard deviations from the mean are infrequent, the head circumference percentile should be compared with the percentiles for height and weight in order to detect a relative microcephaly or macrocephaly. (The latter may uncover a mild case of Dandy Walker cyst, which can present as school failure.) In addition to seizures and dysarticulation, Bax and Whitmore (1973) noted a high incidence of squint and undescended testes in children with later learning problems (cf. Stewart et al., 1966). Although not clinically useful, dental abnormalities are more common in children with MBD than in normal controls (H. J. Cohen and Diner, 1970; H. J. Cohen, Diner, and Davis, 1975; Goodwin and Erickson, 1973).

A large variety of minor malformations can be observed in children with hyperkinesis. Lerer (1977) noted that simian creases and Sydney lines were two to three times more frequent in hyperactives than in control children. Hart et al. (1974) found minor stigmata in 11.3% of MBD subjects compared to none in controls. Children with diffuse brain damage exhibited a 40% incidence of "microsymptoms of Mongolism": epicanthus, malformed pinna, palatal underdevelopment, nasion hypoplasia, clinodactyly, syndactyly, palmar Macacus line, and a large gap between the first two toes (Daryn, 1961). A scoring system for 18 such anomalies (Table 9) has been extensively researched in various pediatric populations. A number of surveys and prospective studies document a significant correlation between a high anomaly score and:

1. A hyperactivity cluster (hyperkinesis, impulsivity, impatience, intractability, inability to delay gratification, nomadic/frenetic play, perseveration) in males (Firestone, Lewy, and Douglas, 1976; Halverson and Victor, 1976; Quinn and Rapoport, 1974; Waldrop and Goering, 1971; Waldrop and Halverson, 1971; Waldrop, Pederson, and Bell, 1968)
2. A hypoactivity cluster (hypokinesis, overconcentration, withdrawal, shyness, timidity, stubbornness, inhibition) in females (Halverson and Victor, 1976; Waldrop and Halverson, 1971)
3. Clumsiness (Waldrop and Halverson, 1971)
4. An increased incidence of obstetrical and perinatal complications (Quinn and Rapoport, 1974; Rapoport et al., 1977)
5. A history of paternal hyperactivity (Quinn and Rapoport, 1974; Quinn et al., 1977)
6. Infant irritability within the first year of life (Quinn et al., 1977; Rapoport et al., 1977)
7. The presence of a learning disability or a severe emotional disturbance (but not with a neurosis) (Steg and Rapoport, 1975)
8. Higher plasma levels of dopamine-β-hydroxylase (DBH) (Rapoport, Quinn, and Lamprecht, 1974; Rapoport et al., 1977)

Employing the same stigmata score on a population of first graders, Rosenberg and Weller (1973) found no correlation with performance IQ (draw-a-person test), motor ability (Porteus Maze Test) or classroom behavior; there was a low inverse correlation with verbal intelligence (Peabody Picture Vocabulary Test) and a strong inverse correlation with global academic performance.

Table 9.   Minor physical anomalies

Head
1. Fine electric hair
    Won't comb down   2
    Soon awry after combing   1
2. Two or more hair whorls   0
3. Head circumference
    > 1.5 SD   2
    $< 1, \leq 1.5$ SD   1

Eyes
4. Epicanthus
    Lacrimal caruncle wholly covered   2
    Lacrimal caruncle partially covered   1
5. Hypertelorism
    Inner canthal distance > 1.5 SD   2
    Inner canthal distance $> 1, \leq 1.5$ SD   1

Ears
6. Low set
    Helix > 0.5 cm below naso-orbital line   2
    Helix < 0.5 cm below naso-orbital line   1
7. Absent lobule
    Lower border of ear oblique   2
    Lower border of ear horizontal   1
8. Malformed   1
9. Asymmetrical   1
10. Soft and pliable   0

Mouth
11. High-arched palate
    Roof of mouth steepled   2
    Roof of mouth high, flat, and narrow at top   1
12. Furrowed tongue   1
13. Geographical tongue   1

Hands
14. Curved fifth finger
    Marked clinodactyly   2
    Slight clinodactyly   1
15. Simian (single transverse palmar) crease   1

Feet
16. Long third toe
    Longer than second toe   2
    Equal to second toe   1
17. Partial syndactyly (webbing) of two middle toes   1
18. Large gap between first two toes   1

Adapted from Waldrop and Halverson (1971) with permission. Items 1, 3, 4, 5, 6, 7, 11, 14, and 16 significantly differentiated schizophrenics from normal children and were weighted 1 or 2. Items 8, 9, 12, 15, 17, and 18 were more frequent among schizophrenic children and were weighted 1. Items 2, 10, and 13 are additional anomalies weighted 0. One may calculate a total count (maximum 18 anomalies) or a weighted score (maximum 24); the correlation between these two is better than 0.9. Standards for inner canthal distance may be found in Feingold and Bossert (1974). For more detailed descriptions (including photographs, drawings, and normative data), see Waldrop and Halverson (1971).

Physical anomaly scores appear to be stable from infancy through elementary school (Quinn et al., 1977), with no black/ white differences (Waldrop and Goering, 1971). Between two and four anomalies can be expected in the general population (Waldrop et al., 1978), but scores of five or more are considered significant (Quinn et al., 1977; Quinn and Rapoport, 1974). If one uses stigmata scores to screen for behavior and learning problems, there will be few false positives but many false negatives (Waldrop et al., 1978). This last observation, together with the fact that physical anomalies do not correlate with soft signs, suggests that these stigmata are indexing a specific subgroup (or subgroups) of the MBD population with certain types of insults to the fetus in the first trimester. The same minimal genetic or traumatic insult that causes these anomalies subtly and permanently influences catecholamine metabolism. These minor malformations thus reflect a specific organic component in disorders of behavior and learning in childhood, and they can serve as clinical markers for minor deviations in the embryogenesis of the central nervous system.

HANDEDNESS, LATERALITY, AND DOMINANCE

Let not thy left hand know what thy right hand doeth.

Matthew 6:3

Orton (1928, 1937, 1966) noted a high incidence of left-handedness in children presenting with delayed speech, stuttering, clumsiness (developmental apraxia), and problems in reading, writing, and spelling. More recent studies have not confirmed this association. L. Belmont and Birch (1965), for example, found a 10% rate of sinistrality in both good and retarded readers, and Clark (1970) reported similar reading levels for both right- and left-handed students. Kinsbourne (1975) suggested that although there was no support for a causal relation with sinistrality, there might yet exist a statistical association with certain subgroups of learning-disabled children. Left-handedness, however, may only seem to be a factor in learning disabilities because it may contribute to the selection of which of a population of equally involved learning-disabled children actually get referred for medical evaluation: if the teacher interprets sinistrality as a sign of organic brain pathology, left-handers will find themselves overrepresented in medical surveys.

Failure to establish hand preference by 2 years of age should be considered suspect. The association of mixed handedness or incomplete hand dominance with dyslexia has been documented by A. L. Benton and Sahs (1968) and Ingram and Reid (1956). Less than 20% of normal and almost 50% of reading-disabled 7-year-olds exhibit mixed hand dominance (A. J. Harris, 1970). Thus incomplete handedness is much more strongly related to learning problems than is sinistrality. Kucera's laterality quotient:

$$LQ = \frac{R + \frac{A}{2}}{R + L + A}$$

can be employed when using a series of tests for handedness; R, L, and A are the number of tasks performed with the right, left, and both hands, respectively. A score between 75 and 100 indicates right-handedness; a score below 50, left-handedness; and a score in between, mixed handedness (Kosc, 1974). The more detailed a protocol one uses for assessing handedness, the more likely one is to uncover some degree of mixed handedness. The Harris Tests of Lateral Dominance (A. J. Harris, 1970) demonstrate excellent clinical applicability.

The significance of mixed eye-hand-foot preferences (crossed motor patterns) is more problematical. A number of researchers have fairly conclusively demonstrated that crossed laterality (e.g., left-eyed, right-handed, and left-footed) has no relationship to either the diagnosis or treatment of reading problems (Cashdan, Pumfrey, and Lunzer, 1971; Ginsburg and Hartwick, 1971; Rabinovitch et al., 1956; A. A. Silver, 1961). For example, L. Belmont and Birch (1965) found consistent eye-hand dominance in half of both average and retarded readers, with mixed eye-hand dominance being present in just under a third of both groups (cf. Figure 15). The concept of a dominant eye is debatable from a neurological standpoint (Bettman et al., 1967; L. J. Lawson, 1968; Money, 1966b); eyedness may simply indicate which eye has the least refractive error and be totally unrelated to cerebral asymmetries (Benson and Geschwind, 1968).

If laterality refers to the child's awareness of the two sides of his body and his ability to identify them as left and right, then directionality refers to the ability to project this laterality onto the outside world (A. J. Harris, 1970). Thus most children, by 5 years

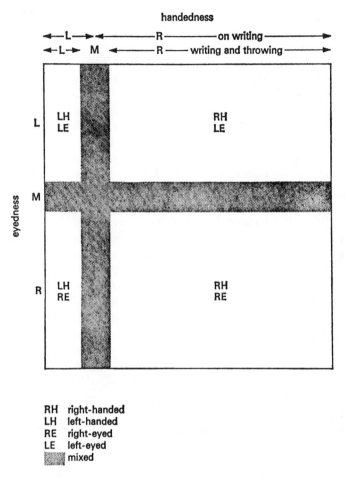

handedness

RH   right-handed
LH   left-handed
RE   right-eyed
LE   left-eyed
▨   mixed

Figure 15. Handedness and eyedness. When considering crossed eye-hand later-ality as related to learning disability, it must be noted that only 61% (in this popu-lation of 1,544 children) of subjects have their preferred hand and eye on the same side. (From M. M. Clark, *Reading Difficulties in Schools,* Penguin Books, Balti-more, © 1970, M. M. Clark, reprinted with permission.)

of age, can tell the examiner which is their right and which is their left hand; by 7 years of age they can perform crossed commands like "Put your right hand on your left ear" or "Put your left hand on your right knee." It is often not until 9 years of age that a child can identify right and left on a mirror image; e.g., "Place your right hand on my left knee" (with the examiner sitting facing the child). More than two mistakes in a dozen trials can be considered deficient. (Some Catholic school teachers will make the sign of the cross in the Greek manner—right and left reversed—when facing an entering first grade class.) Poor right-left discrimination for age has been strongly associated with reading retardation (Ginsburg and Hartwick, 1971; A. A. Silver, 1961) and lower performance IQ scores (L. Belmont and Birch, 1965). For example, at 7 years of age almost 40% of reading-disabled children exhibit directional confusion compared to 5% of controls (A. J. Harris, 1957).

The right-left confusion and the mixed handedness observed in dyslexia probably reflect conceptual deficiencies in spatial orientation—symbolic problems in labeling otherwise intact perceptions (A. J. Harris, 1970; Rabinovitch, 1962; Schroeder et al., 1978). (Delayed handedness tends to be associated with lower *verbal* IQs.) Thus right-left disorientation is not a perceptual dysfunction to be treated but simply another manifestation of a basic underlying verbal deficit.

Difficulties with handedness, laterality, and directionality have frequently been interpreted within the context of a hypothesis of increasing lateralization of *brain* function. Asymmetry certainly reflects a higher level of information processing than a more primitive bilateral symmetry (Bateson, 1972, 1979). But the relationships between cerebral dominance and peripheral manifestations of lateralization are fairly complex and still largely unknown (Touwen, 1972). Both handedness and brain lateralization appear to occur much earlier than previously thought and are probably preprogrammed (Kinsbourne, 1975; Levy and Levy, 1978; Rudel, Teuber, and Twitchell, 1974). Developmental trends in human functional asymmetry are not easily demonstrated; even handedness may be detected in early infancy (Caplan and Kinsbourne, 1976; Hiscock and Kinsbourne, 1978). While recent research is documenting a significant correlation between cerebral dominance and learning disabilities, it must be remembered that the common clinical tests for handedness, laterality, and directionality bear little or no proved relationship to cerebral dominance.

ELECTROENCEPHALOGRAPHY

The EEG has exercised a fascination in the field of learning disabilities out of all proportion to its actual contribution. Its imagined ability to "diagnose" brain damage was so influential a decade ago that many school systems required an EEG report before special class placement. As an instrument for the localization of dysfunction, its accuracy is greatly inferior to that of the electrocardiogram (EKG) for cardiac disorders; its specificity even for seizure disorders is only fair to good. False positives and false negatives range between 10% and 20%. In addition, the pediatric EEG demonstrates striking changes with age, so that there is no single set of reference norms; the expertise required for a clinically useful EEG interpretation on a learning-disabled child is relatively rare. Outside a specific research protocol, the routine ordering of an EEG on MBD/SLD children should be discouraged. Nevertheless, after its limitations are recognized, the EEG may play an important role in the understanding of disorders of learning and behavior in children.

The EEG findings common in MBD/SLD are frequently described as mild, questionable, or age-related abnormalities: diffuse, posterior and occipital slowing (associated with immaturity), generalized defects of organization (lack of rhythmicity), focal transient sharp waves, and poor development (decreased amplitude) (Charlton, 1972; Klinkerfuss et al., 1965; Klonoff and Low, 1974; Satterfield, 1973; Schain, 1975). Children with nonverbal disturbances have more abnormal EEGs, and Myklebust (1973) suggested a greater probability of electrocortical dysfunction with predominant right hemispheric involvement. Muehl, Knott, and Benton (1965) noted that the more severely learning disabled tended to have the more normal EEGs. The subgroup of slow learners with borderline intelligence and diffuse brain involvement would presumably exhibit the more obvious electrical disturbances. On the other hand, Satterfield, Cantwell, Saul, and Yusin (1974) found the more abnormal EEGs among the hyperkinetic children with higher IQs. The positive EEG findings in MBD children do tend to normalize over the succeeding decade (Hechtman, Weiss, and Perlman, 1978).

Power spectral analysis of the EEG shows greater intrahemispheric coherence (uniformity and synchronization of electrical activity) in dyslexic and hyperkinetic children in contrast to greater interhemispheric coherence in controls (Montagu, 1975; Sklar, Hanley, and Simmons, 1972). Satterfield et al. (1972) and Satterfield, Cantwell, and Satterfield (1974) have proposed that the excessive slow wave activity demonstrated by power spectral analysis along with decreased skin conductance levels and immature evoked cortical responses (see below) all support the hypothesis that the MBD child's primary problem is one of underarousal. The same methods of computerized analysis suggest that drug responders are characterized by higher mean resting amplitudes and wider ranges of resting amplitudes.

The reported incidence of mild EEG abnormalities is approximately 40% to 50% in MBD and 15% to 30% in controls (Capute, Niedermeyer, and Richardson, 1968; Hughes, 1971; Klinkerfuss et al., 1965; Klonoff and Low, 1974). Hughes (1971) claimed to be able to correctly classify 77% of underachievers by visual inspection of the EEG. If one accepts an EEG abnormality rate of 50% for MBD and 20% for normals along with a 10% incidence of MBD, then given a population of 10,000 children, the EEG would correctly classify 500 of the 1,000 MBD subjects and misclassify 1,800 of the 9,000 normal children. Although this would yield a 77% overall success rate, for every normal child who did not receive an EEG the percent would decline toward 50%.

For a considerable period of time, 14 and 6 per second positive spikes (ctenoids) were considered pathognomonic for MBD. Studies of normal populations demonstrated that ctenoids are found in approximately 20% of normal children, with a peak incidence in early adolescence (Demerdash, Eeg-Olofsson, and Petersen, 1968; Lombroso et al., 1966). Although nowhere near as diagnostic as was once hoped, the 14 and 6 phenomenon may actually be slightly more common in the learning-disabled population. It is a valid conclusion that there are no specific EEG correlates for MBD, learning disability, or dyslexia (A. L. Benton and Bird, 1963; Klonoff and Low, 1974). The EEG signs frequently reported as characteristic of these syndromes are in the same category as soft neurological signs and need to be subjected to the same discriminating clinical scrutiny. Attempts to correlate EEG findings directly with intellectual and academic performance have been even less rewarding (Hartlage and Green, 1973; Hughes, 1968).

The posteriorly prominent alpha (α) rhythm (8–13 cycles per second) is an index of relaxed wakefulness. The α attenuation response refers to the decrease in α when attention is paid to a stimulus (Fuller, 1978; Shetty, 1973). In MBD/SLD children the α that is present tends to be poorly organized, with larger amplitudes at rest and longer latencies and weaker arousal responses (less α attenuation) to stimuli (Grünewald-Zuberbier, Grünewald, and

Rasche, 1975). Stimulant medication normalizes α activity and synchrony in drug responders (Martinius and Hoovey, 1972; Shetty, 1971, 1973). These EEG findings are consistent with a lowered state of arousal and an attention deficit in MBD.

A procedure that never achieved wide acceptance is the Photo-Metrazol Activation Test. Photopentylenetetrazol is injected during an EEG recording with a stroboscopic light-flashing stimulus. The end point of the test is the dose (mg/kg) of drug necessary to produce a specific cortical seizure discharge on the EEG. Effective low dosages theoretically reflect diencephalic dysfunction—an insufficient shielding of the cortex from irrelevant stimuli. Hyperkinetic children thus exposed to intense storms of unscreened stimuli can have their photometrazol threshold raised by amphetamines (Laufer et al., 1954; Laufer, Denhoff, and Solomons, 1957). This midbrain screening deficit hypothesis dovetails into the previous hypoarousal/attention deficit theory if one identifies the diencephalic filtering device as the neural system that is underaroused or hypofunctioning.

EVOKED RESPONSES

Computer technology has combined with the EEG to enable the study of averaged evoked cortical responses with both visual and auditory stimuli. In general the visual-evoked responses (VER) of MBD/SLD children are immature; they resemble the responses of younger normal children. The VERs of MBD/SLD subjects demonstrate longer latencies and larger amplitudes. Latencies presumably reflect the speed of information processing; since they decrease with age, longer latencies represent immature responses. Larger amplitudes result from greater synchronous activity of underlying brain areas and therefore possibly greater attention (Njiokiktjien, Visser, and de Rijke, 1977; Shields, 1973). Conners (1974a) reported that stimulant medication had little effect on VER amplitudes but it significantly decreased latencies in drug responders. Buchsbaum and Wender (1973) used evoked responses to predict clinical response to drugs; with an intense stimulus, evoked responses diminished in responders on drugs and were augmented in nonresponders on drugs (cf. Greenhill et al., 1973). However, successful prediction using this method obtained only a 64% accuracy. Lux (1977) suggested that hemispheric differences in VERs might measure hemispheric dominance. Halliday et al. (1976) cautioned that the attentional state (active or passive) was critical to the discrepancies among many reported studies. Preston, Guthrie, and Childs (1974) and Preston et al. (1977) demonstrated significant amplitude differences between dyslexics and controls in VER components over parietal and left angular gyrus areas; these differences were marked for semantic stimuli but present even for nonsemantic stimuli. They concluded that the relationship between the VER and reading was reliable and detectable but marginal and of limited diagnostic utility in individual cases.

In the auditory-evoked response (AER; in the literature this abbreviation sometimes refers to the averaged evoked response, whose stimulus may be either auditory or visual), latency decreases and amplitude increases with age (Ohlrich and Barnet, 1972). Satterfield, Lesser, Saul, and Cantwell (1973) and Satterfield (1973) characterized the AERs of MBD children as immature, with decreased amplitudes and increased latencies compared to age-controlled normal subjects. The data of Pricher, Sutton, and Hakerem (1976) on AERs obtained under different attention conditions added support to the hypoarousal theory of MBD: they also demonstrated a normalizing effect of stimulant medication on AER differences. In what is probably the most impressive application of EEG technology to date John et al. (1977) used a complex neurometric battery to discriminate learning-disabled from control children with greater accuracy than psychometric tests. Abnormal EEG or AER asymmetry was present in 88% of learning-disabled subjects and in only 8% of controls. It was also possible to profile different types of learning disorders using this neurometric battery (Figure 16).

The latest advance in electroencephalographic technique is the brainstem auditory-evoked potential (BAEP) (Galambos and Hecox, 1978; Figure 17). In a preliminary study, Sohmer and Student (1978) found that MBD children had longer brainstem transmission times (interpeak latencies), suggesting delays in information processing.

In the debate over the importance of EEG findings in MBD/SLD children it must be kept in mind that EEG abnormalities do not necessarily implicate an exclusively structural etiology. The significance of EEG abnormalities needs to be distinguished from any discussion of causation. Approximately 50% of children with nonspecific emotional and behavioral disorders have abnormal

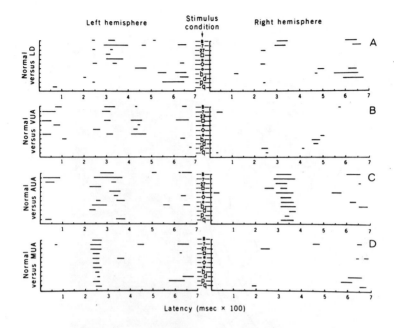

Figure 16. Auditory-evoked responses: neurometric battery. The graphs on the left show the differences for all combined left hemisphere electrode placements and those on the right show the right hemisphere differences. In each graph the horizontal bars indicate the significant ($p < 0.01$) latency responses for each of the 11 different stimulus conditions in the neurometric battery (NB). Clear spatiotemporal differences in auditory-evoked responses (AERs) exist between the normals ($N=20$) and each of the differentially disabled children: LD, learning disabled ($N=30$); VUA, verbal underachievers ($N=10$); AUA, arithmetic underachievers ($N=10$); MUA, underachievers in both verbal and arithmetic skills. Each group is characterized by a distinctive spatiotemporal pattern. (From E. R. John et al., Neurometrics, *Science 196*, pp. 1393-1410, copyright ©1977 by the American Association for the Advancement of Science, with permission.)

BEAM, the mapping procedure devised by Duffy, Burchfiel, and Lombroso (1979), may facilitate the visual display of this kind of data.

EEGs (Aird and Yamamoto, 1966). This may reflect a mixture of: 1) behavioral disturbances with a contributing organic substrate, and 2) cerebral electrical patterns whose development has been disturbed by the influence of an abnormal early environment (cf. Stevens, Sachdev, and Milstein, 1968). On the other hand, a normal EEG reading does not rule out organic brain involvement: certain brain areas can be presumed to be electrically silent with current techniques "since some cerebral structures are less eloquent than others" (Capute et al., 1968). The EEG in all its modal-

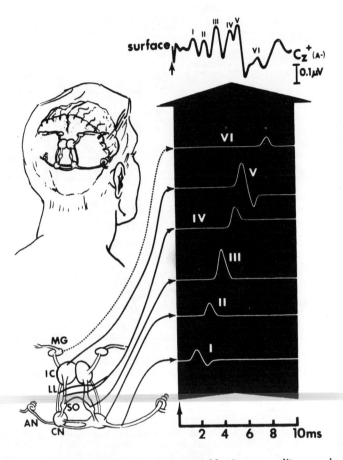

Figure 17. Oversimplified version of sequential brainstem auditory-evoked potential (BAEP) generation and volume conduction to surface electrodes. Composite response (top right) BAEPs probably originate primarily from axonal projections of the indicated nuclei rather than from the nuclei themselves. Click stimulus is indicated by the arrow and BAEPs are plotted C_z positive-up or earlobe (A) negative-up. AN, auditory nerves; CN, cochlear nuclei; SO, superior olives; LL, lateral lemnisci; IC, inferior colliculi; MG, medial geniculates. Evidence for the thalamic origin of wave VI is circumstantial. (From J. J. Stockard, J. E. Stockard, and F. W. Sharbrough, Nonpathologic factors influencing brain stem auditory evoked potentials, *American Journal of EEG Technology 18*, pp. 177–209, © 1978, with permission.)

ities has at present little to contribute to the understanding of individual patients. It offers, however, electrophysiological support for certain theoretical constructs, and as the analysis of subgroup patterns is further refined, the newer EEG technologies have the potential for achieving relevance to individual case studies.

DRAWING TESTS

A variety of different drawing tests is available for the office evaluation of the learning-disabled child (Figure 18). They help in the assessment of fine motor abilities, visual-perceptual motor (VPM) skills, and a number of higher-order cognitive processes. While all of the following tests show some relationship to learning disabilities, they correlate poorly with one another and are therefore probably measuring distinct aspects of the complex act of VPM integration. As with soft signs, minor malformations, and subtest scatter, deviations on these tests neither diagnose nor exclude learning disabilities; rather they present the physician with information that needs to be clinically interpreted and integrated into a comprehensive assessment of the whole child.

The *Gesell figures* (Figure 18A) present the classic series of figures to copy. With this, as with all drawing tests, it is imperative for the examiner to observe the child's performance instead of just leaving him to copy the drawings on his own. By 3 years of age most children will copy a circle with recognizable accuracy, and by 5 years of age right-handed children will draw the circle with a counterclockwise motion. This transition to a predominantly counterclockwise direction is not observed in Israeli children (Goodnow, 1977), so there does appear to be a significant cultural contribution to this developmental trend. Obviously this clockwise/counterclockwise orientation must be observed in action since it is in no way apparent on the finished product. With the "Union Jack" figure, most children under 5 years of age fill in the rectangle with horizontal lines that do not cross the midline; between 5 and 6 years of age some slanting diagonals cross the vertical midline; and after 6 years of age two diagonals and a horizontal line cross a vertical midline (Ames, 1968a). Here again, the child's reconstruction of the figure must be observed; some learning-disabled children will draw eight superimposed triangles (or pie slices), while others will extend eight radii from a center point in the rectangle. Many times these deviations in conceiving the gestalt of the figure cannot be discovered in the final product. Like errors on many other tests, problems in figure copying are susceptible to many different interpretations. Cerebral palsied

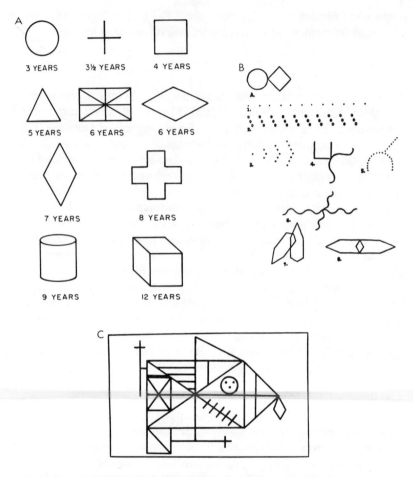

Figure 18. Commonly used drawing tests. A, Gesell figures. (Adapted from Taylor, 1961.) B, Bender-Gestalt Test. (From L. Bender, *A Visual Motor Gestalt Test and Its Clinical Use,* 1938, American Orthopsychiatric Association, New York, with permission.) C, Rey-Osterreith Complex Figure. (From A. Rey, *Test de Copie et de Reproduction de Mémoire de Figures Géométriques Complexes,* 1959, Les Editions du Centre de Psychologie Appliquée, Paris.)

children have trouble with such designs because of movement deficits and associated problems in spatial perception (Abercrombie, 1968). With other types of brain injury, the source of the difficulty may lie in a generalized immaturity of cognitive function or in conflicting orders and associated movements, reflecting more localized damage (Abercrombie, 1970). When the child's copy bears little resemblance to the original, he should be asked to comment on this discrepancy in order to ascertain whether he actually perceives the difference. Poor figure copying has not been related to any specific pattern of learning disability, although Park (1978) showed a tendency for reading-disabled children with fewer difficulties on figure copying to exhibit more sequencing errors in reading.

The *Draw-a-Person* (DAP) test, first standardized by Goodenough (1926), has been shown to correlate with mental age (D. B. Harris, 1963; D. B. Harris, Roberts, and Pinder, 1970). Significant distortions, suggestive of a learning disability, may lower the estimate of intelligence based on this test by itself. A. A. Silver and Hagin (1967) noted a peculiar downward displacement of the arms and a slanting position of the DAP figure on the page in dyslexic subjects, and other patterns of errors have been reported in children with learning problems (Table 10). Nevertheless, there are no specific deviations on the DAP characteristic of children with learning disabilities. Kindergarten experience has remarkably little effect on the DAP scores of children between 5 and 7 years of

Table 10. Signs of organicity on the Draw-a-Person test

Signs in young children	Signs in adolescents
1. Omission of body	1. Gross maturity of drawing
2. Arms not in two dimensions	2. Poor integration of parts
3. Arms not pointing down	3. Emptiness of facial expression
4. Arms incorrectly attached	4. Lack of details
5. Hands absent	5. Omission of parts, especially neck
6. Legs not in two dimensions	6. Transparent or absent clothing
7. Pupils absent	7. Flattened heads
8. Neck absent	8. Displacement of extremities
9. Incorrect number of fingers	9. Petal-like or scribbled fingers and toes
10. Less than two pieces of clothing	

The column for young children is from Koppitz (1968); items 1–6 are significant for children 6 years of age and older; items 7–10 are not significant until 7 years of age. The column for adolescents is from Schildkrout, Shenker, and Sonnenblick (1972).

age; certain items appear to be more influenced by early school experience—two dimensions on arms and legs, more than one piece of clothing, the correct number of fingers—but the overall scores are in the same range (Koppitz, 1968). The idea that early scribbling will influence later reading ability (Baker and Kellogg, 1967) must still be considered speculative. Particularly stylized drawings that seem out of keeping with the child's performance on other tests should be repeated a little later in the evaluation; a "rote" performance on this task would be suggested by a carbon copy repetition of the previous drawing. The DAP may also be used to indicate the general emotional state of the child (DiLeo, 1970, 1973); especially helpful in this regard is the kinetic family drawing (KFD), in which the child is requested to draw a picture of his entire family with everyone doing something (Burns and Kaufman, 1970, 1972). An interpretation of these drawings (aided by questioning the child) is usually fairly straightforward.

The *Bender-Gestalt* (B-G) test has received the most evaluation as a test for children with learning disorders. Whereas most children complete the nine figures in about 6 minutes, MBD children tend to finish faster—in approximately 4 to 5 minutes (Koppitz, 1975). Abnormal B-G performances may correlate with abnormal electroencephalograms (cf. Koppitz, 1975). As with other drawing tests, a marked discrepancy between the child's mental age and his drawing age is more suggestive of a learning disability. Longitudinal evaluations of VPM with the B-G does not demonstrate "catch-up"; learning-disabled children persist in immature levels of performance on this task (Koppitz, 1975; Figure 19). The test appears to accurately reflect school readiness in middle to lower class children while underestimating the performance of children with a higher SES (Koppitz, 1963).

A. A. Silver (1950) recommended the Gesell figures, the DAP, and the B-G as the basic drawing battery for use by the pediatrician. The *Rey-Osterreith Complex Figure Drawing* (Rey, 1959; Figure 18C) should be added since it appears to reflect some distinct organizational abilities. Originally designed as a memory test for adults with head injuries, perseveration and poor organization on this task have been interpreted as signifying frontal lobe damage (Lhermitte, Deroulsne, and Signoret, 1972). Osterreith (1944) has described the qualitative evolution of children's approach to this test; the order in which subjects draw the different parts can be permanently recorded by having the child use a de-

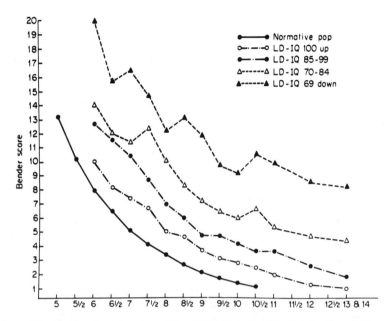

Figure 19.   Bender-Gestalt scores. (From E. M. Koppitz, *The Bender Gestalt Test for Young Children, Vol. II,* © 1963, Grune & Stratton, New York, with permission.)

fined sequence of colored pens. It is interesting to observe children successfully complete the Gesell figures and then experience a lot of difficulty with this complex figure that is actually composed of the same shapes; perhaps this is similar to what happens with the child who reads single words in isolation but fails when presented with the same words on a page of print. Examples of drawing performance by learning-disabled children are presented in Figure 20.

VISUAL AURAL DIGIT SPAN (VADS) TEST

Short-term memory is frequently tested utilizing such tests as digits forward (DF), digits reversed (DR), and sentence memory. In addition to an age level, which can be found on these items in the Stanford-Binet, the Wechsler Intelligence Scales for Children (WISC), and other tests, qualitative deviance may be noted when the child remembers all the numbers but juggles the sequence,

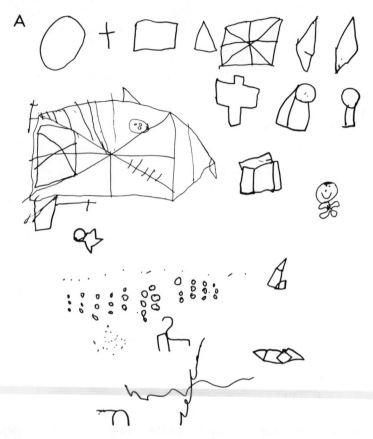

Figure 20. Drawings by learning-disabled children. A, This 6-year, 3-month-old boy was completing first grade with resource room help; all his drawing scores were within 1 year of his chronological age.

when the child obtains a better score for digits backward than for digits forward, or when the child makes peculiar substitutions in the sentences.

Rudel and Denckla (1974) have suggested that the child whose performance on DF is worse than on DR has left hemispheric involvement (i.e., a language component to his learning disability); conversely, the child whose DR score is worse has right hemispheric involvement (i.e., a visuospatial component to his learning disability). Inability to repeat any digits at all is probably a sign of bilateral hemispheric involvement. Since the DR

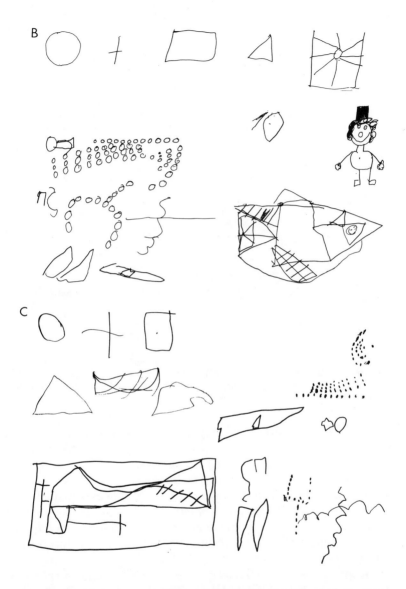

Figure 20. B, This 9½-year-old girl is best described as an overfocused over-achiever; she was doing grade-appropriate work at the cost of 3 to 4 hours of home-work a night. Her drawings appear more immature than those of the previous child (A). C, This 7½-year-old boy had a history of chronic hearing impairment associated with repeated myringotomies and P-E tube placements in early child-hood. In addition to language delay, however, he also demonstrated a perfor-mance IQ lower than his verbal IQ.

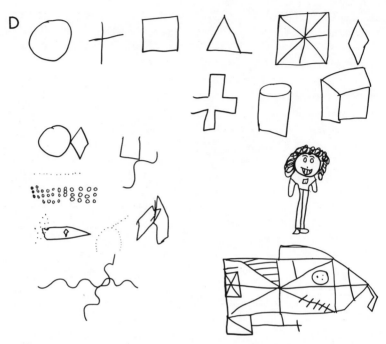

Figure 20. D, This 9½-year-old girl exhibited hyperactivity and impulsivity with no evidence of a learning disability. (The original drawings covered four to five sheets of paper; the size relationship has not been held constant between the different sets of drawings.)

score shows a greater tendency to improve with age, the digit span discrepancies lessen over time for left hemisphere-involved children and increase for right hemisphere-involved children. Performance on digit span tests can be impaired by anxiety, but only by transient anxiety (A state) and not by stable personality trait anxiety (A trait) (Hodges and Spielberg, 1969); thus the anxiety that interferes with digit memory should be immediately apparent to the clinician administering the test and not deduced from poor performance on the test.

Koppitz (1977) has devised a very useful variant of the digit span test, the Visual Aural Digit Span (VADS) test. In the four subtests of this instrument, digits forward are assessed, with the numbers being presented and reported both orally and in writing: Aural-Oral (AO), Visual-Oral (VO), Aural-Written (AW), and Visual-Written (VW). Additional subscores may be obtained for Aural Input (AO+AW), Visual Input (VO+VW), Oral Expression (AO+VO), Written Expression (AW+VW), Intrasensory Integration (AO+VW), and Intersensory Integration (VO+AW). The time for administration and the difficulty of interpretation for this test are roughly equivalent to those of the Bender-Gestalt test. The task involved in this test is scholastically relevant (as opposed to many neuropsychological items, which are totally outside the child's experience) and psychiatrically neutral (many reading-disabled youngsters find letters and words emotionally laden). VADS subscores give hints of intra- and intersensory processing difficulties at a practical level that the physician may then compare with the results of the more detailed psychoeducational evaluation. Although VADS scores improve with age, the delays seen in learning-disabled children do not catch up; indeed, they even fall relatively farther behind over time (Figure 21). Digit memory tests thus appear to measure some complex, higher-order processes with an organic basis.

EDUCATIONAL ASSESSMENT

The pediatrician performs visual and auditory perceptual tests to give himself sufficient insight into how this particular child processes information so that the doctor can better interpret the formal psychoeducational evaluation and intelligently support either the school system's recommendation for placement or the parent's challenging the appropriateness of this placement. The child's performance on these tests may also be used as a starting point to counsel parents on how to understand and manage their child's behavior. At the very least, the neurodevelopmental profile should not be diametrically opposed to the results of the school's evaluation. The pediatrician will always need to supplement his impression by a formal psychometric assessment since he is susceptible to a "halo effect," in which single characteristics color the overall judgment (Heim, 1970). This distortion in perspective is even more likely in the child with uneven cognitive development.

Since academic underachievement is the sine qua non of learning disability, it is important for the pediatrician to estimate the child's educational level. (The underachievement should never be assumed on the basis of perceptual test deficits.) Detected patterns of underachievement may be diagnostically significant. The

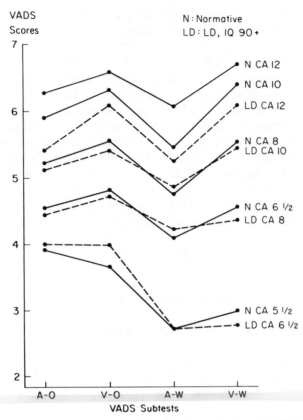

Figure 21. VADS subtest scores in normal and learning-disabled children. VADS subtest patterns for learning-disabled (LD) children resemble the VADS subtest pattern seen in younger normal children. Thus, the scores for 6½-year-old LD subjects approximate those of normal 5½-year-olds; 8-year-old LD children have scores similar to 6½-year-old normals; 10-year-old LDs are similar to 8-year-old normals; and after 12 years of age LD children (2½ years behind the normative sample) showed no further improvement. Another way of interpreting these VADS profiles for LD children is to view them as demonstrating a fairly stable VADS quotient (between 80 and 85) with a tendency to plateau early (cf. Appendix B). (From E. M. Koppitz, The Visual Aural Digit Span Test, © 1977, Grune & Stratton, New York, with permission.)

child who has already mastered basic literacy and computational skills in the first half of elementary school and who then has trouble with subjects like social studies or science may have problems with motivation or individual teachers. On the other hand, the child who from the beginning of grade school experiences difficulties in acquiring the basics of reading and mathematics is suspect for SLD. Striking discrepancies between reading and arithmetic grade levels suggest dyslexia or dyscalculia.

The child who is not detected as learning disabled until the fourth grade has probably used good decoding skills to survive; when comprehension becomes more prominent he begins to fail. The child with poor word recognition (decoding) skills tends to be identified much earlier. Analogously, a child may do well in arithmetic computations in the first three grades but begin to fail when "word problems" are introduced in the fourth grade. Ingram et al. (1970) charged that educational attainment tests were unreliable before the third grade; the child with good rote skills will score spuriously high on such instruments. It is important to realize that the commonly used Wide Range Achievement Test (WRAT) for reading is solely a measure of single word recognition (decoding) and not of comprehension.

Thus the pediatrician performs academic screening tests to determine: 1) which subject areas are involved, 2) whether a reading problem is one of word recognition or comprehension, and 3) whether mathematical deficits are computational or reasoning in nature. The physician may also informally try to correct the child's errors in order to see how he responds to teaching (A. J. Harris and Roswell, 1953; Sapir and Wilson, 1978).

PARENT COUNSELING

To give good advice is absolutely fatal.

Oscar Wilde

MBD/SLD is not a disorder of one season, but a lifelong handicap that assumes varying manifestations throughout development. From a hyperactive fetus to a colicky, difficult infant with little regularity to his schedule; to a hyperkinetic, clumsy preschooler with poor peer relationships; to a learning-disabled school age child with increasing frustration and secondary behavior problems; to an illiterate, unemployable teenage dropout—this dismal progress may seem inevitable with certain children. Before graduating from high school, the MBD/SLD child will go through four to six school placements, each with different principals and guidance counselors; his teachers will change annually. Individual psychoeducational assessment/counseling through the school system will probably not occur more frequently than every 2 years. The pediatrician is the only professional able to provide the necessary continuity to the kind of counseling that the family with a learning-disabled child will need. It is essential that the doctor acquire the necessary training and expertise in developmental disabilities to assume this responsibility.

While the pediatrician discusses his findings within the context of brain damage, he will qualify them as not conclusively diagnostic. In exploring the parental response to an organic component to their child's problems, the most frequent response found is one of relief. Even without reinforcement from others, parents often spontaneously assume guilt for having mismanaged their child and caused his difficulties. The realization of a biological contribution can free the parents from an overemphasis on emotional factors and enable them to focus their energies more constructively (cf. Clements and Peters, 1962; Erenberg, 1973; M. D. Hertzig et al., 1969; Willerman, 1973). But at the same time that he accents the position of MBD on the brain damage spectrum, the pediatrician must also stress the essential normality of the child. The very process of a multidisciplinary assessment may inadvertently highlight all the child's negative behaviors, his deficits and weaknesses; the psychopathology of everyday life is capable of overinterpretation. To compensate for this tendency a deliberate effort should be made to have the parents describe the child's good qualities, his strengths and assets, those moments that make him a joy and pleasure to his family (cf. Bryan and Bryan, 1975). These positive aspects help put the brain damage model in a proper perspective.

A helpful analogy is to compare the behavior and learning problems. If reading is a difficult achievement for the MBD/SLD child, social learning is even more difficult to acquire. Whereas a teacher will carefully analyze the child's reading errors, just as careful a dissection needs to be applied to the child's behavioral faux pas. "Social imperception" is one of the hallmarks of the MBD/SLD child (D. J. Johnson and Myklebust, 1967) and, in the long run, perhaps the most disabling. Parents are the ideal managers of their child's social learning problems, but they could use help. Stimulant medication only makes the child more receptive to teaching. The pediatrician must familiarize himself with the techniques of behavioral psychology; many families that describe the children as uncontrollable and unaffected by any mode of discipline can benefit from parent training workshops in behavior modification (Dubey and Kaufman, 1978). Several individual counseling sessions are frequently necessary; it is rare that parents will be significantly helped by merely reading a book or two on behavior management. Two of the best volumes for parents are by R. S. Lewis, Strauss, and Lehtinen (1960) and S. L. Smith (1978); Gardner's (1966, 1973) books may help children toward a better understanding of their problems.

While parents should be encouraged to work on the child's social learning, they should be discouraged from tutoring the child in areas of academic weakness (cf. A. J. Harris and Roswell, 1953); at the most they can help the child with homework when specifically instructed to do so by the teacher. While this may help relieve stress within the family, after-school tutoring by nonfamily members should also be discouraged. With appropriate class placement, the learning-disabled child should not need to spend many more hours per day on academic work than the normal child. In selected cases, peer tutoring may be well received (Dineen, Clark, and Risley, 1977), and sometimes tutoring *by* the learning-disabled child may reinforce his own academic accomplishments.

Some general guidelines for parents include: 1) avoid failure and frustration; 2) prepare the child for change when necessary but try to minimize change by keeping the home on as organized a routine as possible; 3) reduce distractions and irrelevant cues in learning situations; 4) keep discipline consistent (Conners, 1967; Erenberg, 1973; Schmitt, 1977). Finally, the pediatrician may have to remind the parents that: 1) "teacher" does not imply a specialist in child development or child psychology, and 2) it is unsafe to assume the teacher is a potential ally against the system (Melton, 1975).

Thomas Alva Edison, Auguste Rodin, George Bernard Shaw (with his phonetic spelling errors), and William Butler Yeats are among the notable persons who suffered from learning disabilities (Illingworth and Illingworth, 1966). With delayed and deficient language skills, behavior problems, and poor school performance, Albert Einstein gave evidence even in his later visually mediated, creative thought of a dominant hemisphere deficit (Patten, 1973). Napoleon's spelling difficulties may have been influenced by his bilingual childhood, but his worsening dysgraphia (possibly contributory at Waterloo) suggests a more pervasive disorder. Hans Christian Andersen was a poor student who never did achieve spelling accuracy (Table 11), yet he created tales of an almost pain-

Table 11. Hans Christian Andersen's spelling errors[a]

MANSCHESTER	NORD KENT RAILROOD	BRACKFEST	SCHAKSPEARE
REVENTLAU	LINDOA	GIOFFRY	SIDNY SCHMIDT
DAVISTOCK	DAVIDSTOCK	LUNGH	RODINDENDRON
MONT BANK	TAMPS	TEMPS	PUNSCH
RUSSEL PLACE	SATURDAI	IERROLD	CITTY
MARRY	ROSCHESTER	KHATEDRAL	HENRIK
BULWOR	STROH	CAP	SCHACKSPEAR
LUNZ	LUNG	CHRISMAS CAROLS	HOUSCHOLDS WORD
MACKBETH	MACHBETH	STANFJELD	

From Critchley (1963) by permission.
From M. Critchley, The problem of developmental dyslexia, *Proceedings of the Royal Society of Medicine 56*, pp. 209–212, © 1963, with permission.
[a]Made in his diary of his London visit in 1857.

ful beauty and sensitivity. Many schools today, even knowing of a child's problem, would persist in scoring such misspellings though the composition were as lyrical as one of Andersen's. Caution must be exercised when using such success stories to reassure parents; modern technological society is more regimented and unyielding in "paper" requirements. For example, in the past the field of medicine attracted a large number of bright dyslexic and dysgraphic individuals; as medical school admissions committees come to rely more heavily on standardized multiple-choice examinations, fewer SLD children may gain entrance to this profession. While undergraduate programs have attempted to make allowances (cf. Admissions Testing Program, 1978; Gollay and Bennett, 1976), the same cannot be said for graduate-level programs.

PSYCHO-PHARMACOLOGY

Drugs promise neither the passport to a brave new world nor the gateway to the inferno. Properly employed as a single component of a total treatment program, they can be helpful in realizing the goal of the healthy development of children.

Eisenberg (1971)

Amphetamines were first used in the treatment of hyperactivity more than 40 years ago by Bradley; since that time the popular conception of the action of such stimulant medications on hyperkinetic children is that they exert a paradoxical calming effect on behavior. Although there is still some debate over a sedative effect (Montagu and Swarbrick, 1975), it is now generally accepted that psychostimulants do not demonstrate a paradoxical but rather a typical energizing effect on inhibitory systems (Barkley, 1977). It thus appears that the critical factor for determining the drug's effect on behavior is the child's initial level of arousal and attention (see Figure 22). It is, therefore, not surprising that, using low doses (0.5 mg/kg) of amphetamine, Rapoport et al. (1978) found that *normal* preadolescent boys exhibited decreased motor activity, decreased reaction time, and improved performance on cognitive tests.

The basic pharmacological mechanisms for the action of amphetamines include: 1) the release of catecholamines (norepinephrine and dopamine) from sympathetic nerve terminals, 2) inhibition of the re-uptake of released catecholamines, and 3) blocking the enzymatic degradation of catecholamines by monoamine oxidase (MAO) (Figure 23). Since catecholamines are the predominant neurotransmitters in the reticular activating system (arousal and attention), the limbic lobe (appetitive and drive states concerned with the reinforcement of learning), the diencephalon (screening stimuli from cortical awareness), and the basal ganglia (motor coordination), drugs that alter the levels of these neurotransmitters (especially if this alteration is selective for specific pathways) can be expected to have profound effects on attention, activity, motor coordination, and learning.

When stimulant medications like dextroamphetamine (Dexedrine) and methylphenidate (Ritalin) are given to hyperactive children, the overall rate of behavioral improvement ranges between two-thirds and three-quarters of the cases: 64% (Denhoff, Davids,

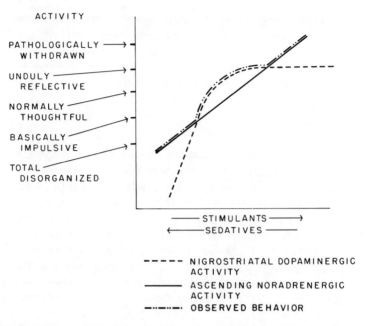

ACTIVITY

PATHOLOGICALLY ——→
WITHDRAWN

UNDULY ——————→
REFLECTIVE

NORMALLY
THOUGHTFUL

BASICALLY
IMPULSIVE

TOTAL
DISORGANIZED

——— STIMULANTS ———→
←———SEDATIVES ———

- - - - - NIGROSTRIATAL DOPAMINERGIC
ACTIVITY
——————— ASCENDING NORADRENERGIC
ACTIVITY
—··—··—· OBSERVED BEHAVIOR

Figure 22.   The neurochemical modulation of activity level may be viewed as reflecting a balance between the regulatory nigrostriatal dopaminergic system and the ascending ventral noradrenergic pathway (possibly in association with the mesolimbic dopaminergic tract). That the effects of amphetamines are inversely related to the amount of pretreatment motor activity has been noted in mice (Glick and Milloy, 1963) and humans (Millichap and Johnson, 1974). (After Humphries et al., 1979; Kinsbourne and Caplan, 1979; and P. Wender, 1971.)

and Hawkins, 1971), 72% (Lerer, Lerer, and Artner, 1977), 79% (Schain and Reynard, 1975), 70% (J. Swanson et al., 1978), 78% (Sleator and von Neumann, 1974), 81% by teacher report and 64% by parental report (Wolraich, 1977), and 75% (Barkley, 1977, reviewing 110 studies on 4,200 hyperactive children). Differences between teacher and parent behavioral ratings are frequent and may be due to: 1) giving medication only early in the day so that the effects wear off by the time the child comes home from school, 2) the parents dealing with the child on a more one-to-one basis, or 3) a differential susceptibility to a placebo effect. The difficulty in trying to compare the results of various drug studies stems from: 1) slight (but probably significant) differences in the diagnostic criteria for entrance into the study, 2) marked heterogeneity of outcome variables—from telephone interviews to extensive formal reassessment, and 3) a broad spectrum of severity often re-

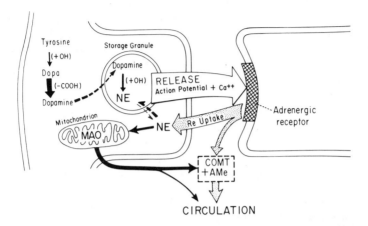

PRESYNAPTIC NEURON   POSTSYNAPTIC NEURON

Figure 23. Catecholamine synapse. Neurotransmitters are released into the synaptic cleft from storage vesicles. Inactivation is by: 1) re-uptake into pre-synaptic neuron, 2) intraneuronal monoamine oxidase (MAO), and 3) extraneuro-nal catechol-O-methyl-transferase (COMT) with its cofactor, S-adenosylmethi-onine (AMe). Amphetamines work by mimicing catecholamines at receptor sites, impairing re-uptake, and inhibiting MAO activity (Snyder and Meyerhoff, 1973). (From R. J. Baldessarini, Pharmacology of the amphetamines, *Pediatrics 49,* pp. 694-701, © 1972, American Academy of Pediatrics, with permission.)

flected in the source of the subject population—with the milder cases being found in private practice and the more severe (and possibly drug-resistant) cases being referred to specialty clinics (cf. Wolraich, 1977).

A commonly accepted description of the action of psycho-stimulants is that they influence behavior positively without enhancing learning (Rie et al., 1976). Minimal brain dysfunction (MBD) children on medication demonstrate increased attention span, concentration ability, and alertness along with decreased activity levels, distractibility, and impulsivity (Barkley, 1977; Conners et al., 1969; Schain and Reynard, 1975; Wolraich, 1977). That the decreased hyperactivity is not a sedative effect is evidenced by the increased vigilance, persistence, and level of free-field activity (Stroufe and Stewart, 1973). The improved behavior does not occur in isolation: Humphries, Kinsbourne, and Swanson (1978) observed an increase in mother-child cooperation on a specific task, and Sprague and Gadow (1976) noted greater social interaction between teacher and child, both in the treatment condition. General behavioral improvement is, however, rare in the pre-school-age population: hyperactivity can be decreased in this group only at the cost of a fairly negative effect on mood and peer relations (Schliefer et al., 1975). With an overall success rate of 10% in this age group, stimulants should be used with caution before the beginning of school. It is not known whether this low rate is due to greater diagnostic confusion attendant on diagnosing organic hyperkinesis in younger children or whether it is secondary to an age-related difference in neurotransmitter balance.

The most frequently used instrument to monitor behavioral response to medication is the Conners Abbreviated Teachers Rating Scale (CATRS; see Conners, 1969), in which a score from 0 (not at all) to 3 (very much) is applied to the following 10 items:

1. Restless/overactive
2. Excitable/impulsive
3. Disturbs other children
4. Short attention span
5. Fidgety
6. Distractible
7. Easily frustrated
8. Cries often/easily
9. Mood lability
10. Temper tantrums/unpredictable behavior

Total scores range from 0 to 30, with 15 being 2 standard deviations above the mean. An even simpler instrument is the Global Teacher Scale, in which behavior is assessed as:

1. Very much improved
2. Much improved
3. Minimally improved
4. No change
5. Minimally worse
6. Much worse
7. Very much worse

This brief rating correlates very well with the CATRS (Sleator and von Neumann, 1974; Sprague and Sleator, 1973).

Behavioral ratings are probably more susceptible to a placebo effect than are other, more objective measures. Thus Lerer et al. (1977) reported a 2% incidence of positive response to placebo when handwriting was the outcome measure, but a 14% placebo

response on a behavioral instrument. In a study of chlorpromazine, Werry et al. (1966) noted a 50% minimal improvement on
placebo, a 20% placebo response similar to that of the treated
group, and a 20% incidence of side effects in the placebo group.
Using methylphenidate and a placebo, Knights and Hinton (1969)
found that 37% of placebo children improved on a parent rating
scale and 67% of placebo children improved on a teacher rating
scale (despite these high placebo effects, this study still demonstrated a significant drug effect). Schain and Reynard (1975) were
able to keep their placebo response rate down to 2% by screening
out overtly disturbed families. While placebo response presents a
significant obstacle to the interpretation of group studies, in the
analysis of drug effects in individual cases it should play a much
less prominent role. The medication being used is technically not a
placebo—it is not pharmacologically inert, and a good proportion
of nonresponders can be expected to demonstrate adverse (or
overdose, if the drug is pushed far enough) reactions (cf. Figure
22). Perhaps the most distinguishing clinical characteristic of placebo responses is that they do not last.

While there are no studies to show that medication produces
any *permanent* improvement in learning, there are an increasing
number of reports of significant short-term effects on cognitive
processes. Stimulant medication produces improved paired-associate learning; improved performance on the Porteus Mazes,
achievement tests (especially arithmetic), and perceptual tests
(Draw-a-Person, Frostig, auditory synthesis); and enhanced rote
learning (Conners et al., 1969; Millichap et al., 1968; Wolraich,
1977). When Epstein et al. (1968) noted an increased performance
IQ with a decreased verbal IQ, they attributed the latter to a
depressant effect of medication. Such changes in verbal and performance IQs are quite variable and probably more reflective of
sample heterogeneity (Conners, 1971). When learning-disabled
children without accompanying behavioral disorders are given
stimulant medication, they exhibit improved psychological test
scores and unchanged achievement test scores (Gittelman-Klein
and Klein, 1976).

Global test score differences tend to be positive but low, with
no single test consistently demonstrating drug effects (Knights,
1974). Laboratory measures of learning, on the other hand, have
achieved a much greater degree of consistency, but their practical
relevance to classroom performance and behavior remains moot.

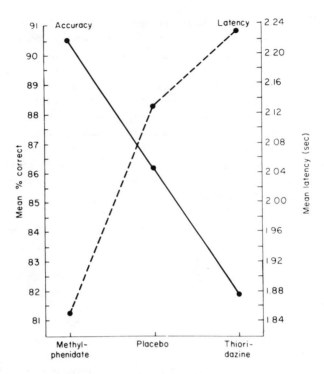

Figure 24.   Accuracy and latency curves for three drug conditions. Compared to controls (placebo), methylphenidate increases accuracy and decreases latency; thioridazine demonstrates the opposite responses. (From R. L. Sprague and J. S. Werry, Methodology of psychopharmalogical studies with the retarded, in N. R. Ellis (ed.), *International Review of Research in Mental Retardation,* © 1971, Academic Press, New York, with permission.)

Using a paired-associate learning task (a short-term memory test), Sprague, Barnes, and Werry (1970) demonstrated that stimulant medication both decreased reaction time and increased the percentage of correct responses; phenothiazines presented the opposite set of responses and must therefore be considered highly inappropriate therapy for children with learning disabilities (Figure 24). Sprague and Sleator (1973, 1977; cf. Brown and Sleator, 1979) also reported different dose response curves for different target behaviors: enhancement of (paired-associate) learning was maximal at 0.3 mg/kg of methylphenidate and began to decline at 0.4 mg/kg; social behavior continued to improve up to doses of 1.0 mg/kg (Figure 25). Since social behavior is the target measure tapped by

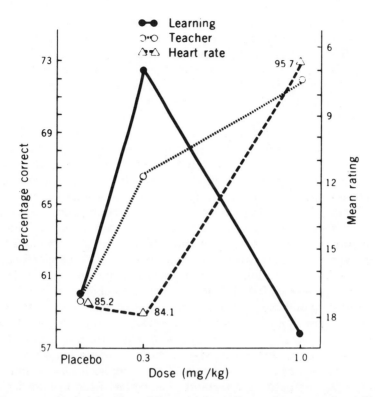

Figure 25. Methylphenidate: differential dose effect on learning and social behavior. Learning was enhanced at a methylphenidate dose of 0.3 mg/kg but inhibited at the higher dose of 1.0 mg/kg; social behavior (as assessed by teacher ratings) continued to improve when the dose was increased to 1.0 mg/kg. Physiological side effects were also noted at the higher dose. (From R. L. Sprague and E. K.
Sleator, Methylphenidate in hyperkinetic children, *Science 198,* pp. 1274–1276,
© 1977 by the American Association for the Advancement of Science, with permission.)

most rating scales, these authors raise the possibility that the
commonly employed dosages of stimulant medication may be in-
terfering with learning. It must be cautioned, however, that laboratory learning is far from synonymous with classroom learning
(Kolata, 1978). Millichap et al. (1968) reported average doses of 1.5
mg/kg/day; Schain and Reynard (1975) suggested an optimal dose
range of 0.2 to 1.9 mg/kg. Kinsbourne and associates have used
another paired-associative task to document the state-dependent
nature of learning in hyperactive children: both the facilitation of
learning and the long-term retention of learned material are con-

tingent upon the drug state, and the total time hypothesis was supported only in the drug state (Dalby et al., 1977; J. Swanson et al., 1978; J. Swanson and Kinsbourne, 1976). In the near future such laboratory measures of learning may allow more objective clinical discrimination of drug responders from nonresponders as well as titration of the dosage, to minimize any inhibitory effects on learning.

In addition to their positive effects on behavior and cognition, stimulants also affect motor coordination and motor skill acquisition (Wade, 1976). Knights and Hinton (1969) reported an average increase of 11.4 points on the Wechsler Intelligence Scales for Children (WISC) performance IQ (with most notable increments on Coding, Picture Completion, and Block Design), along with improved motor coordination and perceptual-motor skills; Schain and Reynard (1975) noted frequent improvements in speech and handwriting on medication. Humphries et al. (1979) logically attributed motor coordination improvement to increased attention. However, Lerer et al. (1977) demonstrated that both the improved handwriting and the rapidly improved performance on soft neurological signs (jerky saccads, finger-to-nose, rapid alternating movements, mirror movements, and choreiform movements; Lerer and Lerer, 1976) were independent of the drug's effect on behavior and attention. If one recalls: 1) the complex interweaving of catecholamine pathways through the region of the median forebrain bundle with some tracts being concerned with affective behavior, others concerned with the focusing of attention, and still others with aspects of fine motor coordination, and 2) the delicate chemical balance among the similar if not identical neurotransmitters subserving all these functions within a microscopic area, then both the frequent association and frequent dissociation of drug effects becomes more understandable, if not quite intelligible.

SIDE EFFECTS

The pharmacological effects of amphetamines include (peripherally) an increase in blood pressure, dry mouth (secondary to mucosal vascular constriction), relaxation of bronchial musculature, and (centrally) anorexia (loss of appetite), insomnia (wakefulness), and decreased fatiguability. Between 10% and 20% of children on stimulant medication will experience at least transient side effects, such as anorexia, insomnia (more prominent with dextroamphetamine), irritability, headache, depression, excessive crying, gastrointestinal disorders, abdominal pain (more common with methylphenidate), urticaria, increased heart rate/pulse, and elevations of blood pressure (diastolic with methylphenidate and systolic with dextroamphetamine (Epstein et al., 1968; Erenberg, 1972; Knights and Hinton, 1969; Winsberg et al., 1974). Some children may develop the "amphetamine look," a pale, pinched, serious facial expression with dark hollows under the eyes (Laufer, 1971; Laufer and Denhoff, 1957). Hallucinations from dextroamphetamine and delirium, ataxia, dyskinesia, and psychosis from methylphenidate are all self-limited conditions; they disappear upon withdrawal of the drug (Winsberg et al., 1974). Stimulant-induced dyskinesias are characterized by facial tics, lip smacking, grimacing, and choreoathetoid and dystonic movements of the extremities; they are idiosyncratic reactions (similar to those observed with phenothiazines) that can occur with normal doses. Methylphenidate can interfere with the enzymatic degradation of a number of anticonvulsants, thus causing serum levels to rise to toxic levels (Garrettson, Perel, and Dayton, 1969).

Safer, Allen, and Barr (1972) first reported a relative decrease in height and weight on dextroamphetamine and methylphenidate. Annual height increments were three-quarters of normal; annual weight increments were two-thirds of normal. Dextroamphetamine inhibited weight more than methylphenidate, but the rebound that occurs when the drugs are discontinued was greater for dextroamphetamine (Safer and Allen, 1973; Safer, Allen, and Barr, 1975). Beck et al. (1975) and Oettinger, Gauch, and Majovski (1977) found no significant effect of long-term stimulant medication on growth; Gross (1976) noted a slight decrease over the first 3 years of treatment, with a maximum effect in the first year and a reversal of the effect in later years, so that by final follow-up, not only was there no stunting but rather an overall increase in height and weight. Millichap (1978) noted that the annual growth rate was greater than normal in two-thirds of his patients on medication and he questioned whether stimulants might enhance growth. Oettinger et al. (1974) and Schlager et al. (1979) found a delayed bone age in MBD children. Finally, Aarskog et al. (1977) reported that growth hormone-releasing factor was modulated by dopaminergic neurons and that both dextroamphetamine and methylphenidate were potent growth hormone stimulants. Between alterations in growth hormone homeostasis and delays in bone age, long-term predictions of effects on height and weight are difficult to make. However, even the largest magnitudes for long-term growth suppression/enhancement do not appear to be of such a size as to warrant withholding of medication when indicated (cf. Roche et al., 1979).

A last potential side effect that needs to be considered is the possibility of drug abuse. Clinical experience with other groups of children on long-term medication (e.g., insulin) does not suggest a higher incidence of later drug abuse, but rather the opposite. Children who depend on chronic medication seem to develop earlier a more mature attitude toward drugs. In young adults 10 years after initial stimulant therapy, Laufer (1971) found no evidence of drug abuse—only 9% had experimented with drugs, and none was addicted. In another study, adolescents who had been treated with stimulants showed a 10% incidence of drug abuse and a matched control group showed a 37% incidence (Beck et al., 1975). Hechtman et al. (1976) also reported a higher incidence of drug abuse in control adolescents.

It is usually assumed that most children outgrow the need for medication in adolescence (Denhoff et al., 1971); thus Laufer (1971) reported that hyperactivity disappeared in 61% of subjects between 12 and 16 years of age. Systems that were previously delayed may mature or alternative means of control may be developed as the child grows older. Sleator, von Neumann, and Sprague (1974) found that within 2 years of starting stimulant medication, one in four drug responders no longer needed medication. But although symptomatology may lessen or change, not all children outgrow the need for medication in adolescence. Mackay, Beck, and Taylor (1973) pointed out that adolescence and pubescence did not necessarily correlate with neurological maturation (cf. Figure 26). Lerer and Lerer (1977) found that 16 out of 27 MBD adolescents demonstrated subjective and objective improvement on methylphenidate. Arnold, Strobl, and Weisenberg (1972) tried stimulant medication on a previously untreated adult with a history suggestive of MBD; the patient experienced decreased anxiety and increased concentration, self-esteem, and depression. Thus the subtle but pervasive effects of MBD that persist into adulthood may respond to medication.

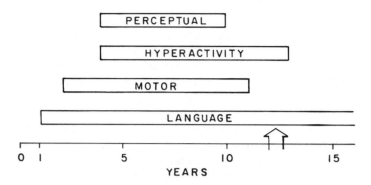

Figure 26. Although the onset of puberty (arrow) does not necessarily indicate full central nervous system maturation, it does frequently coincide with a sufficient degree of neurological development that medication may no longer be necessary. The bars indicate the degree of expression of various types of symptoms with age. Thus perceptual-motor disorders may become obvious in the preschool child but are rarely apparent by the middle of elementary school; hyperactivity usually becomes noticeable just before the onset of formal schooling and persists into early adolescence. Motor clumsiness is usually noted in the toddler and tends to improve dramatically in the late elementary grades; although the sequence is far from invariant, this motor improvement is frequently followed within 1 to 2 years by the adolescent growth spurt, and then by a marked spontaneous remission of hyperkinetic symptomatology so that medication can then be withdrawn. In some form (language delay, dysarticulation, reading disorder, or speech dysfluency), language involvement persists through the entire life-span of the (MBD)/specific learning disability (SLD) child.

OTHER DRUGS

In addition to dextroamphetamine, methylphenidate, and pemoline, numerous other drugs have been employed with learning-disabled, MBD children. In general such drugs come from the field of child psychiatry, where they have been used for severely disturbed children, or from the field of pediatric neurology, where they have been used to treat seizures. The research data to support their efficacy is much less than those for the psychostimulants and in some cases is little more than anecdotal. Levoamphetamine succinate (Cydril) is actually an amphetamine; it has a lower euphoric potential and produces much less anorexia. It takes about 3 weeks to observe a drug effect; the medication is available in a time-release capsule (Arnold and Wender, 1974). Deanol (Deaner) has produced an equal number of reports demonstrating and failing to demonstrate any effect on hyperactivity

(Millichap and Fowler, 1967); given the paucity of experience, it is not recommended. Imipramine is an antidepressant with a structure very close to the phenothiazines; its efficacy is similar to methylphenidate and may be considered an alternative drug for nonresponders (Gittelman-Klein, 1974; Quinn and Rapoport, 1975). Chlorpromazine (Thorazine) is a phenothiazine that is much less effective than dextroamphetamine (Greenberg, Deem, and McMahon, 1972); Werry et al. (1966) claimed that the reduction in IQ on this drug is not drastic. Hydroxyzine (Atarax) is ineffective (Greenberg, Deem, and McMahon, 1972), but haloperidol (Haldol) shows some positive effects (Werry, Aman, and Lampen, 1976). The use of this latter butyrophenone in the pediatric age group should, however, be restricted to cases of Gilles de la Tourette syndrome (multiple tics, barking, and coprolalia). Lithium carbonate appears to be of little use (Greenhill et al., 1973). Amitriptyline hydrochloride is an antidepressant with mild tranquilizing properties. Yepes et al. (1977) reported that it improved attention as well as parent and teacher ratings of hyperactivity and aggression, but it had no effect on short-term memory or impulsivity. Rossi (1967) proposed using it in combination with methylphenidate since it reversed the anorexia caused by that drug. Even if there were evidence to suggest that amitriptyline prevented the putative growth suppressant effect of methylphenidate, it would be hard to defend administration of double psychotropic medications to children.

The association of behavior disorders with learning disabilities frequently raises the question of an occult seizure disorder. If in addition there is a history of aggressive or violent outbursts, the possibility of a temporal lobe seizure disorder will be raised. But temporal lobe seizures are almost unheard of in the primary grades and extreme caution must be exercised before interpreting minor EEG abnormalities (so common in MBD/SLD children) as subclinical seizures (cf. Denhoff, 1976; M. E. Olson, 1975). The anticonvulsant phenobarbital is a sedative that "paradoxically" stimulates and worsens the behavior of MBD children (Millichap, 1973); the possibility has been mentioned before that the other common anticonvulsants may deleteriously affect learning. Millichap et al. (1969) have, however, reported paroxysmal seizure discharges (especially in the temporal area) to be inversely correlated with scores on subtest 6 of the Detroit Test of Learning Aptitudes, a test of auditory perception; the scores improve with diphenylhydantoin therapy. Whether this represents a definable subgroup, possibly related to certain types of acquired aphasia, awaits further investigation.

Schnackenberg (1973) first suggested that caffeine, the stimulant in coffee, might supplement the effect of methylphenidate on hyperactivity. Firestone et al. (1978) and Huestis, Arnold, and Smeltzer (1975) found only insignificant improvement with pure caffeine. Using whole coffee, Harvey and Marsh (1978) demonstrated significant improvements of concentration, digit span, visual-motor coordination, and parent/teacher rating scales, and Firestone et al. (1978) noted some improvement in impulsivity and general behavior. These preliminary studies with caffeine suggest that: 1) as a nonspecific stimulant, caffeine does affect the systems involved in MBD positively (see Figure 22), and 2) the magnitude of the effect seen with caffeine renders it an unlikely substitute for Schedule II drugs. It would be interesting to learn whether MBD children grow up to be heavy coffee drinkers or whether they should be encouraged to do so.

TREATMENT

There are no characteristics that will definitively identify drug responders before a trial of medication. Conrad and Insel (1967) classified responders as "organics" with three or more of the following: perinatal complications, head injury, convulsions, poor motor coordination, visual-perceptual impairment, subscore scatter, positive neurological findings, EEG abnormalities, and a diagnosis of chronic brain syndrome. Schain and Reynard (1975) found that drug failures tended to have the following characteristics: older than 10 years, a Bender-Gestalt score more than 36 months delayed, a history of infant colic, onset of walking after 18 months, spike discharges on EEG, and obesity. Millichap and Johnson (1974) suggested that the degree of response to stimulant medication was related to the pretreatment level of motor activity and the incidence of abnormal neurological signs. Using heart rate as a physiological measure of attention, Porges et al. (1975) found that children with longer response latencies (i.e., greater attentional deficits) demonstrated more favorable responses to methylphenidate. Satterfield's combining of neurological and electroencephalographic findings to predict drug response is discussed in the section on soft signs.

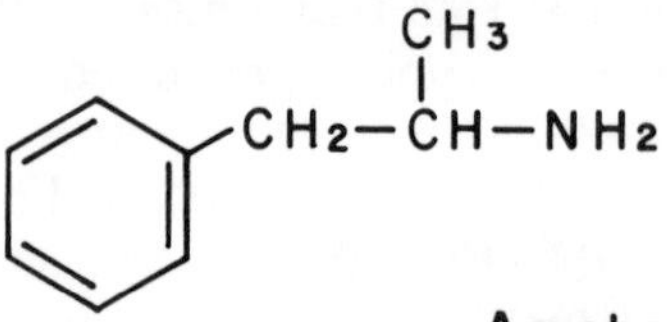

Amphetamine (Dexedrine)

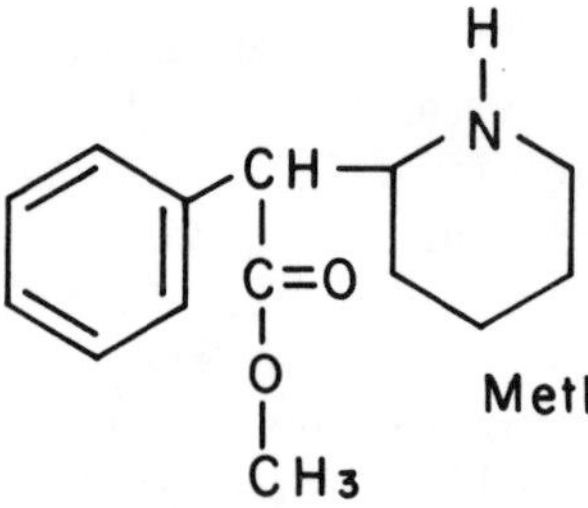

Methylphenidate (Ritalin)

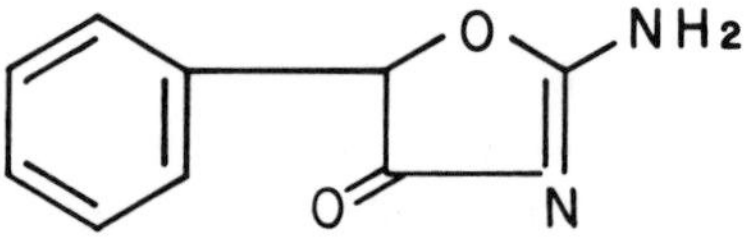

Pemoline (Cylert)

Figure 27. Commonly used psychostimulants. Dextroamphetamine is not recommended for children under 3 years of age, and methylphenidate and pemoline are not recommended for children under 6 years of age because their safety and efficacy in these age groups have not been determined.

With the response to stimulant and other medication being essentially unpredictable, it is possible to spend upwards of 3 years in experimenting with all the different drug forms marketed for hyperactivity. A more rational approach would be to: 1) exclude phenothiazines because of their detrimental effects on learning, 2) not consider, except under rare circumstances, the pharmaceuticals under the heading "other drugs," and 3) become familiar with the dosages and side effects of two of the three most common stimulants: dextroamphetamine (Dexedrine), methylphenidate (Ritalin), and pemoline (Cylert) (Figure 27). This recommendation is not meant to support the "one child, one drug" myth (Fish, 1971); hyperactivity of different etiologies will respond to different medications. Psychostimulants are generally inappropriate for the hyperkinesis associated with mental retardation and severe brain damage; the phenothiazines are usually much more effective. Tranquilizers may be necessary for the hyperactive child with a primary diagnosis of depression or emotional disorder. But clinically the child with MBD/SLD exhibits a high proportion of positive responses to the stimulant category of drugs. Since with the learning-disabled child (as with all the others) the drug therapy is only an adjunct, the greatest effort needs to be directed elsewhere. If trials with appropriate dosages of two stimulants both fail, it would seem to reflect a loss of perspective to continue to vigorously pursue chemotherapy.

Between 1971 and 1973 the proportion of prescriptions for methylphenidate compared to those for dextroamphetamine went from almost equal to two to one (Krager and Safer, 1974). Although Conners (1971) reported fewer side effects with methylphenidate, he admitted that neither drug was superior. L. G. Arnold and Knopp (1973) criticized this myth of the superiority of methylphenidate and pointed out that a small number of patients selectively responded to only one of the two medicines. The Council on Child Health (1975) recommends for the average 6-year-old a starting dose of 5 mg of dextroamphetamine (to a maximum of 40 mg) or 10 mg of methylphenidate (to a maximum of 80 mg) per day; because of the rapid onset of action for these drugs, the dosage may be titrated upward every 2 to 3 days until either an unequivocally satisfactory response or undesirable side effects are achieved. Drug "holidays" for weekends, vacation periods, and summertime are frequently employed to see if the child still needs medication and to allow catch-up growth; however, in view of the pervasive effects of the MBD syndrome on social learning, these are not recommended except briefly once or twice a year to see if the drug continues to be effective. Occasionally with the first month or two of therapy a "tolerance" develops that quickly responds to a minor dose elevation; a further increase in dosage is not usually required until the child undergoes an appreciable change in body size. Where habituation does develop again, Winsberg et al. (1974) recommend alternating two stimulants. Whereas methylphenidate must be taken one-half hour before meals, amphetamines may be taken with or after meals (Kinsbourne and Caplan, 1979; Varga, 1979). Although both of these drugs have a duration of action of approximately 4 hours, effective dose schedules may vary from b.i.d. to q.i.d., with further differences in the size of each dose; such variations may be considered as clinical reflections of different attentional demands for different parts of the day and idiosyncratic fluctuations in the balance of neurotransmitter systems. Insomnia that persists after the first few weeks may actually be helped by a later-afternoon or evening dose. Pemoline offers the advantages of being long-acting, but its initial effects are not noted until after almost a month of treatment, and it takes 48 hours to wear off. In addition to its being fairly time consuming to assess the efficacy of this drug, the absence of a noontime dose at school may inappropriately lessen the school's involvement in a significant component of the child's treatment program. In general, pemoline has no striking advantages and may even be somewhat less effective (Freeman, 1976).

For the pediatrician to reasonably assess whether a medication is working, he needs the cooperation of the child, the parents, and the school. The physician will counsel the parents and the child extensively before instituting a drug regimen and will also contact the school. But if teachers and other school personnel are to take an active professional role in the management of medications for MBD children, they will need far more grounding in the basics of brain-behavior interactions than they currently receive in existing teachers' college programs. It is frustrating for the pediatrician to spend hours dispelling the myths about drug therapy and its role, only to have them resurface in the classroom.

Other factors that need to be considered before the institution of drug therapy include: 1) the costs of the medication and of the follow-up visits necessary to monitor it appropriately, 2) general family stability, common sense, and overall acceptance of the use of medication, and 3) the presence of delinquent adolescent siblings (with a potential for drug abuse) in the home (cf. Solomons, 1973). As to cost, dextroamphetamine continues to run a fraction of the price for an equivalent dosage of methylphenidate. It is an act of therapeutic nihilism to introduce drugs into a chaotic home situation; the parental feedback will be of little help and any positive effects of the medication will tend to get buried beneath the weight of environmental variables.

It has become fashionable in certain circles to criticize the increasing use of stimulant drugs in children as a further example of the medicalization of behavior (Schrag, 1975; Schrag and Divoky, 1975). However, the frequently reported abuse of stimulant medication by indiscriminate overprescribing is often secondary to misinterpretation of data; thus, 5% to 10% of Omaha children were learning disabled but not necessarily on medication (Havighurst, 1976). During the 1970–1971 school year, 2% to 4% of elementary school children in Chicago were on stimulant drugs (Sprague and Gadow, 1976). In a survey of Baltimore schools, Krager and Safer (1974) found that the percentage of elementary school children on psychostimulants increased by almost two-thirds between 1971 (1.07%) and 1973 (1.73%); they also noted that the use of such drugs was more prominent among the affluent. If one accepts the compromise statistic for MBD of approximately a 10% incidence along with a two-thirds significantly positive response to medication, then it would be possible to conclude that on the whole medications were being underprescribed. Abuses (both of over- and underprescription) probably do occur, but epidemiological data are not well suited to document this impression; a more individualized case approach is necessary.

It must be emphasized that, judiciously used, psychostimulants are not constraints on freedom, not chemical straitjackets; treated children are not "jazzed up," and their normal exuberance is not suppressed (Council on Child Health, 1975; Eisenberg, 1972; Erenberg, 1972; R. A. Johnson, Kenney, and Davis, 1976). "The myth that stimulants make hyperkinetic children into conforming robots is arrant nonsense. Restlessness, distractibility, and impulsivity are constraints on freedom, not freedom" (Eisenberg, 1972). Nevertheless, it would appear to be reasonable that any child who specifically refuses drug therapy ought not to have medication forced upon him; parents and physicians should be required to communicate sufficiently with the child to obtain his assent and cooperation.

Drugs are only one part of a comprehensive management program for the child with this chronic neurological handicap; it remains the pediatrician's responsibility to make certain that other treatment modalities are not ignored. It is a rare case—Sleator and von Neumann (1974) reported an incidence of one out of seven for such profound responders in drug successes—where medication alone is all that is necessary to normalize the child's behavior and performance. The recent trend of research to focus on the effects of such drugs on cognition and learning rather than just on behavior should help to discard the charge of mind control; by enhancing cognitive development, psychopharmacology contributes to the achievement of moral autonomy and self-control. If within this perspective drug intervention is unjustified, then, as Broudy (1976) suggested, all intervention, including schooling, is unjustified.

PSYCHOLOGICAL ASSESSMENT: The WISC

How could men be equal in the eyes of God and yet
unequal in the eyes of the Psychologist?

Young,
The Rise of the Meritocracy

Intelligence tests were originally designed to predict academic
performance. They do this better than any other measure; the
global Stanford-Binet IQ still predicts school success more accurately than any of the more recent perceptual- and visual-motor
tests (Bell and Aftanas, 1972). General level of intelligence accounts for a good part of the wide range of academic abilities
found in the classroom. A. J. Harris (1970) reported that the average fourth grade class includes children with reading levels from
grades 2 through 9 (a span of 7 grades); the middle 40% will range
from grades 3.9 to 5.3. Given the essentially normal distribution
of intelligence (Figure 28), 50% of the population will have IQs between 90 and 110, and 66% will have IQs between 85 and 115. In
Harris's typical fourth grade class, therefore, a large part of the
variation in reading levels can be accounted for by IQ alone: for
children with chronological ages 9.2 to 10.2 years (fourth grade
level), the 50% with IQs from 90 to 110 can be expected to have
reading grade levels between 3.1 and 6.0 on the basis of intelligence alone, and the 66% with IQs between 85 and 115 can be expected to have reading grade levels between 2.6 and 6.5. Thus
when Ames (1968b) and Bryan and Bryan (1975) reported that
25% of all children referred for evaluation of learning disability
have IQs below 90, they were highlighting the important contribution of general cognitive level. Similarly, Eisenberg (1966a)
noted that 28% of urban sixth graders were 2 or more years behind in reading, which is within 5% of the percentage predicted
solely from a normal IQ distribution. When a preschool child is referred for evaluation of speech delay, one of the most common
diagnoses is moderate to severe mental retardation; when a
school-age child is referred for evaluation of academic underachievement, one of the most common diagnoses is borderline to
mild mental retardation.

Technically, those children whose academic performance is at
the level expected for their intelligence are not learning disabled;
they are either slow learners or mentally retarded. Although intelligence testing has a high correlation with academic achievement,
it is most useful when there is a discrepancy between IQ and

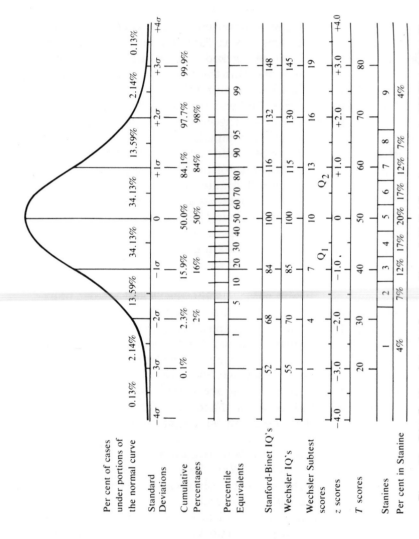

Figure 28. Distribution of standard scores. (From J. M. Sattler, *Assessment of Children's Intelligence*, ©1974, W. B. Saunders Co., Philadelphia, reprinted by permission, Holt, Rinehart & Winston, Inc., New York.)

156

school performance. This is especially true when the discrepancy is marked by a mental age significantly higher than grade achievement levels (Heim, 1970; cf. Appendix B).

On the other hand, the traditional refusal to include children with global IQs between 70 and 85 in the specific learning disorder (SLD) category can be extremely unfair to these children; to describe them as just slow learners may be misleading by failing to take into account their superimposed learning disability, which may in the long run cause them to function more like mildly retarded persons. Similarly, a marked scatter of abilities even in children whose IQs are well within the retarded range may still be interpreted as a superimposed learning disability; the full scale IQ is a poor predictor of these children's progress.

Group tests have no role in the evaluation of specific learning disability. They yield spuriously low IQs for handicapped children (Eisenberg, 1959) whether the child has a reading disorder and is penalized by the written nature of the test or whether he has a short attention span and cannot maintain himself on a task without repeated reinforcement. Therefore all children who, for whatever reason, are suspected of having a learning disability should receive an individual psychometric assessment by a trained child psychologist with experience in testing developmentally disabled children. The importance of such an assessment cannot be overstressed. Intelligence tests were initially designed to objectively describe children's functional levels; they provide for the multidisciplinary assessment the most statistically reliable and valid input data. Unfortunately, capable pediatric psychometricians are in short supply. "Too many consider it to be a menial chore in comparison to the glamour of making Freudian formulations and giving psychotherapeutic advice" (Gofman, 1965). The pediatrician who would rather be doing acute care makes a poor case manager for the chronically neurologically handicapped child; the psychologist who would rather be doing family guidance makes a poor tester.

While the individual psychometric assessment should itself be individualized (Allmond, 1974), the bare minimum is a full Wechsler Intelligence Scale for Children—Revised (WISC-R) (Wechsler, 1974) with all subtest scores reported. By definition, the child with a specific learning disability will have a normal IQ; one needs to be able to assess the unevenness of his performance. A skilled psychologist can tease such information from the Stanford-Binet (Allen and Allen, 1967), but the structure of the

WISC-R makes these findings more accessible to the nonpsychologist team members.

The WISC-R is the test most commonly used in the psychological assessment of learning-disabled children. Its design and the statistical information available on its validity and reliability make it the instrument of choice for this population. Among psychometric tests it best reflects the philosophy that there is no one IQ score for any child but rather a profile of strengths and weaknesses for various psychological abilities. When a child performs very well in one area but poorly in another, the concept of global IQ as an adequate description of that child's potential becomes untenable. The resultant for most interactions between strengths and weaknesses is rarely capable of accurate prediction.

The WISC-R consists of six subtests in the verbal and six in the performance areas to yield 12 subscores and three IQs: a verbal IQ, a performance IQ, and a full scale IQ (Table 12). (In practice, usually only the first five subtests of each group are administered so that the three IQs are based on 10 subscores.) The mean for each of the IQs is 100; the mean for each of the subtests is 15 points; the standard deviation for the subtest scores is frequently taken to be 1.5 (it is actually 3). Thus an IQ range of 70 to 130 corresponds to a subtest range of 4 to 16.

The six verbal subtests are:

1. *Information* The child is asked 30 questions of increasing difficulty, ranging from "How many legs does a dog have?" (easy) to "What are hieroglyphics?" (difficult).
2. *Similarities* "In what way are a ____ and a ____ alike? How are they the same?" Seventeen pairs are presented, ranging from "wheel-ball" (easy) to "salt-water" (difficult).
3. *Arithmetic* This involves 18 problems with simple computations (addition, subtraction, multiplication, and division). After the first four, all are "word problems"; the first 15 are read by the examiner, the last three are read by the child. All are solved mentally.
4. *Vocabulary* "What does ____ mean?" Definitions for 32 common words are requested.
5. *Comprehension* This subtest attempts to measure common sense problem-solving ability with questions ranging from

Table 12. WISC-R subtests

Verbal	Performance
Information (Inf)[L]	Picture Completion (PC)
Similarities (Sim)[L]	Picture Arrangement (PA)[R]
Arithmetic (Arith)[L]	Block Design (BD)[R]
Vocabulary (Voc)[L]	Object Assembly (OA)[R]
Comprehension (Comp)	Coding (Cod)
Digit Span (DS)[L]	Mazes (M)

The L and R superscripts refer to predominantly left and right hemispheric localization, respectively. (See Wechsler, 1974; McFie, 1963; M. J. Meier, 1974; Tarnopol, 1969a.)

"What is the thing you do when you cut your finger?" (easy) to the deontological conundrum "Why is it usually better to give money to a well-known charity than to a street beggar?" Normal-to-high scores on other verbal subtests, such as Information and Vocabulary, along with a low Comprehension score suggests some impairment of judgment.

6. *Digit Span* This assesses the child's ability to repeat increasingly longer sequences of digits both forward and reversed. While all the other verbal subtests rely heavily on previous learning and long-term memory, Digit Span is the only subtest to assess short-term memory.

Arithmetic and Digit Span have the strongest overall correlation with verbal IQ; Information and Vocabulary have the highest overall correlation with general intelligence.

The six performance subtests include:

1. *Picture Completion* Twenty-six drawings, each with one part missing, are presented; the missing parts to be identified range from the mouth on a face (easy) to the shadow of a tree (difficult).

2. *Picture Arrangement* Each of 13 sets of pictures must be arranged to tell a story (such as the commission of a burglary). Whereas Comprehension measures knowledge of social conventions, Picture Arrangement assesses the ability to plan in a social context. A discrepancy between these two subtests may mirror the behavior typical in minimal brain dysfunction (MBD) children where impulsivity prevents the child from utilizing his knowledge of social rules.

3. *Block Design* Nine blocks (each block has two red, two white, and two red and white sides) are arranged to match the patterns on 11 design cards.

4. *Object Assembly* Four jigsaw puzzles are completed to form a girl, a horse, a car, and a face.
5. *Coding* From 5 to 7 years of age symbols are matched to symbols; from 8 to 15 symbols are matched to numbers. A pencil is used to mark the answers.
6. *Mazes* The child must trace a path with his pencil through nine mazes of increasing difficulty.

These last four performance subtests heavily tap visual-motor and perceptual-motor coordination. A. J. Harris (1970) suggested that in those rare cases where one suspects a reading disability to be secondary to emotional disturbance, the perceptual functions measured by these subtests should be unaffected. All of the performance subtests are timed, and half of them include bonus points for speed; arithmetic is the only verbal subtest that is timed. In general, the input on the verbal tests is meaningful, whereas that on the performance tests is not. The functions of the various subtests are presented in Table 13. Intratest variability (or deviance) occurs when the child has difficulty with easy items but then passes more difficult items. While intertest variability is the hallmark of uneven cognitive development, intratest variability may suggest underlying emotional factors (Sapir and Wilson, 1978) but may also reflect cognitive disorders.

V-P DISCREPANCY

The most commonly used WISC diagnostic pattern is the discrepancy between the verbal and performance IQs (V-P discrepancy). Since many of the verbal subtests are considered to have left hemispheric localization and most of the performance subtests to have a right hemispheric localization (see Table 12), the V-P discrepancy may function as a gross index of hemispheric involvement. Thus a lower verbal IQ (impaired left hemispheric function) would be expected in pure reading disorders, whereas a lower performance IQ (impaired right hemispheric function) would be expected in clumsy children without learning disabilities. Rourke, Dietrich, and Young (1973) found such correlations between V-P differences and clinical patterns, but these were seen predominantly in younger children (under 9 years of age). Dykman et al. (1973), on the other hand, reported that V-P differences actually tended to increase with age in learning-disabled children. Learning-disabled children with higher verbal IQs tend to exhibit visuo-

Table 13. Functions if WISC subtests

Subtest	Function	Influencing factors	Subtest	Function	Influencing factors
Information	Range of knowledge Long-range memory	Natural endowment Richness of early environment Extent of schooling Cultural predilections Interests	Picture Completion	Ability to differentiate essential from non-essential details Concentration Reasoning Visual organization	Experiences
Comprehension	Social judgment, social conventionality, or common sense Meaningful and emotionally relevant use of facts	Extensiveness of cultural opportunities Development of conscience or moral sense Ability to evaluate and use past experience	Picture Arrangement	Interpretation of social situations Nonverbal reasoning ability Planning ability	A minimum of cultural opportunities
Arithmetic	Reasoning ability Numerical accuracy in mental arithmetic Concentration Attention Memory	Opportunity to acquire fundamental arithmetic processes	Block Design	Visual-motor coordination Preceptual organization Spatial visualization Abstract conceptualizing ability Analysis and synthesis	Rate of motor activity Color vision
Similarities	Verbal concept formation Logical thinking	A minimum of cultural opportunities Interests and reading patterns	Object Assembly	Visual-motor coordination Perceptual organization ability	Rate of motor activity Precision of motor activity
Vocabulary	Learning ability Fund of information Richness of ideas Memory Concept formation Language development	Early educational environment	Coding	Visual-motor coordination Speed of mental operation Short-term memory	Rate of motor activity
Digit Span	Attention Short-term memory	Ability to passively receive stimuli	Mazes	Planning ability Perceptual organization Visual-motor control	Visual-motor organization

From J. M. Sattler, *Assessment of Children's Intelligence*, © 1974, W. B. Saunders Co., Philadelphia, reprinted by permission, Holt, Rinehart & Winston, New York.

161

spatial errors in reading and spelling, but those with higher performance IQs exhibit predominantly audiophonic difficulties (auditory discrimination, blending, letter-sound association) (Ingram and Reid, 1956). The MBD child with presumably more diffuse brain involvement (bilateral hemispheric) might show little V-P discrepancy but marked subscore scatter. Reitan and Boll (1973) characterized the MBD child with predominantly behavior disorders by a mild decrease in Coding and verbal IQ and the MBD child with academic underachievement by a verbal IQ much lower than the performance IQ. Black (1974) compared children whose V-P discrepancy was less than 10 with children whose V-P discrepancy was greater than 15 points; the latter group had a significant increase in the incidence of hyperactivity, distractibility, visual-perceptual dysfunction, motor clumsiness, abnormal EEGs, and abnormalities of the birth process. But there were no significant differences in academic performance between the two groups. If one uses the V-P difference alone, false positives and false negatives both approximate 40% (Huelsman, 1970). Clark (1970) also found that disabled readers demonstrated the same proportion of marked V-P differences as controls.

Before clinically interpreting the V-P discrepancy, two sets of data need to be considered: 1) the standard error and 2) the normative sample.

Standard error of the estimate (S_{YX}) is a measure of scatter; it is the change in score that can be expected when a child is retested with an equivalent form of the same test. Such changes are the result of chance errors of measurement. Sixty-eight percent of measurements will fall within one S_{YX}; 95% within two S_{YX}, and 99.7% within three S_{YX}. For 7½-year-olds, the S_{YX} for the WISC full scale IQ is 4, for the verbal IQ is 5, and for the performance IQ is 6. Thus if one tests a 7½-year-old child and obtains a performance IQ of 100, the chances are about 68 out of 100 that the range of scores 94 to 106 actually includes this child's true performance IQ (Croxton, 1959; A. J. Harris, 1970; Sattler, 1974).

Many psychologists estimate the average V-P discrepancy score for normal children to be 5 points or less (A. S. Kaufman, 1976b). In the *normative sample* on which the WISC-R was standardized, the *mean* V-P discrepancy was 9.7; 48% of the standardization sample had V-P discrepancies of 9 or more points (significant at the 15% level), 34% had V-P discrepancies of 12 points or more (significant at the 5% level), and 25% had V-P discrepancies of 15 points or more (significant at the 1% level). Therefore, *the average child has a significant V-P discrepancy.* Since such a discrepancy is not an unusual finding, caution should be exercised when relating it to the child's diagnosis (A. S. Kaufman, 1976b).

SUBSCORE SCATTER

Sometimes the discrepancies found between subscores are of greater clinical importance than an observed V-P difference. For example, a child may have a verbal IQ higher than his performance IQ, but the performance subscores are uniformly depressed while the verbal subscores demonstrate an extreme range of scatter. The root of this child's learning problem may be reflected more accurately in the verbal scatter than in the depressed performance scores.

Analysis of WISC subscore scatter does not yield a single diagnostic profile for the learning-disabled child, but several rough patterns do emerge (Table 14). Left hemispheric dysfunction has been characterized as demonstrating Block Design much higher than Vocabulary with depressed Similarities and verbal IQ; right hemispheric dysfunction has been characterized by vocabulary much higher than Block Design, with depressed perfor-

Table 14. WISC subtest patterns

Subtest	Learning disability	MBD	Dyslexia
Verbal			↓
Inf	↓		↓
Sim		↓	
Arith	↓		↓
Voc			
Comp			
DS	↓		↓
Performance		↓	
PC			
PA			
BD	(↑)	↓	
OA		↓	
Cod	↓	↓	↓
M		↓	

Pooled from data and reviews by Ackerman, Peters, and Dykman (1971), Clements and Peters (1962), Huelsman (1970), Kluever (1971), McGlannan (1968), and Owen et al. (1971).

mance IQ and relatively high Similarities (Meier, 1974; Reitan, 1966). Although these patterns are composed of numerical scores, they are best considered as qualitative descriptions of patterns of failure.

Bannatyne (1968, 1974) proposed a recategorization of WISC scaled scores (Table 15); the more severe ("genetic") learning-disabled children have good spatial but poor sequential abilities. Rugel (1974) confirmed that over 40% of learning-disabled children had a pattern of spatial ability that was better than sequential ability (Figure 29). Keogh (1973) also recategorized the WISC subtests and grouped Digit Span, Arithmetic, and Coding (Bannatyne's Sequential Ability) together as reflecting an attention-concentration factor; this factor was significantly low in learning-disabled children. Finally, Vance, Wallbrown, and Blaha (1978) described five WISC-R profiles for reading-disabled children; their Pervasive Language Disability and Distractability syndromes come closest to the patterns reported above.

Again, before clinically interpreting subscore scatter, both standard error and normative sample data need to be considered. S_{YX} for subtest scores for children under 9 years is 1 to 2 points. On the *normative sample* the mean scaled score range (difference between the highest and the lowest scaled scores) was 7 points,

Table 15. Bannatyne's recategorization of WISC subscores

Verbal conceptualization
Sim
Voc
Comp

Acquired knowledge
Inf
Arith
Voc

Sequential ability
Arith
DS
Cod

Spatial ability
PC
BD
OA

From A. Bannatyne, Diagnosis: A note on recategorization of the WISC scaled scores, *Journal of Learning Disabilities 7,* pp. 272–273, © 1974, reprinted by special permission of Professional Press, Inc.

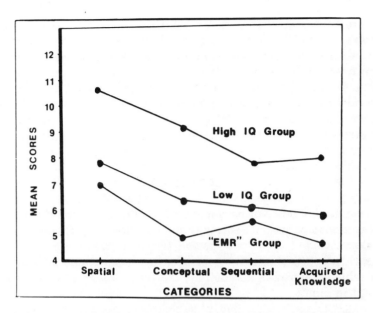

Figure 29. Recategorized WISC-R scores in learning-disabled children. The four factors are from Bannatyne's recategorization of WISC subtests; the high IQ group includes those learning-disabled children with a full scale IQ of at least 76 and a verbal or performance IQ of at least 90; the low IQ group includes those children who did not fit the criteria for the high IQ group, and the "EMR" group is that subgroup of the low IQ group with a full scale IQ below 76. Total $N=208$, with a mean age of 10 years. (From M. D. Smith et al., Recategorized WISC-R Scores of learning disabled children, *Journal of Learning Disabilities 10*, pp. 437–443, © 1977, reprinted by special permission of Professional Press, Inc.)

with a standard deviation of 2. Thus the middle two-thirds of the normal population has a scaled score range between 5 and 9 points. (Many psychologists estimate this range at 3 to 4 points.) A. S. Kaufman (1976a) concluded that if one wanted to consider as significant only scaled score ranges occurring in 15% or less of the normal population, the minimum ranges required would be 7 points on the verbal subtests, 9 points on the performance sub-tests, and 10 points on all the subtests. Alternatively, if one calculates deviation from the mean scaled score, then the 15% level of significance would be obtained only when two (verbal), three (performance), or four (full scale) subtests deviated by 3 or more points from the respective mean scaled scores (A. S. Kaufman, 1976a). The "flat profile" for normal children is a mythical stereotype unsupported by fact. Since the normal child demonstrates quite a bit of subscore scatter (with brighter children showing somewhat more such scatter than duller children), caution must be used if one employs WISC scatter to corroborate a diagnosis of learning disability (cf. Kaufman, 1976a). Subscore scatter generates hypotheses to be tested with regard to the learning-disabled child's functioning (Sattler, 1974). The possibility remains that despite good validity (the degree to which a test measures what it claims to) reported for the WISC subtests, they may not be measuring the relevant deficits in particular learning-disabled children.

CONCLUSION

The infant science of neuropsychology draws on the prestige of its parent disciplines, neurology and psychology, but in reality the intersection of these two disciplines yields results that are still tentative. Although the psychological assessment of learning-disabled children is mandatory, the following points need to be kept in mind:

1. There is no one IQ score for any child; in the presence of significant V-P discrepancy or subscore scatter, the use of the global IQ to measure overall potential is severely limited.
2. Significant subscore scatter may occur in the absence of a V-P discrepancy; therefore, pattern analysis of the subscores is always required.
3. Significant V-P discrepancy and/or subscore scatter may occur in a child without a learning disability and cannot therefore be used to make a diagnosis of learning disability by itself.
4. A child with a severe learning disability may exhibit neither a V-P discrepancy nor subscore scatter; the absence of these findings does not rule out a specific learning disability.

All the above patterns are best considered as cognitive "soft signs"; they suffer from the same limitations as neurological soft signs. In isolation they are high risk to over-, under-, and misdiagnose learning disability. The medical maxim that no sign stands alone must be applied rigorously. Psychological tests are of definite but limited use "as criteria for determining whether central nervous system dysfunction is present or absent. Rather, the tests have more value as descriptive tools of function, as a basis for refining categories of patients and suggesting hypotheses regarding the sources of difference among the observed patterns of functioning, and identifying subgroups who have unique response to therapies" (Conners, 1973).

EDUCATION
AND OUTCOME

Scarcely any area of human activity has been more resistant to scientific analysis and technological change than education.

B. F. Skinner

Education becomes scientific in proportion to the increasing willingness of educationalists to test their hypotheses.

The Saber-Tooth Curriculum

Of all professions, teaching may be characterized as the least scientific and the least accountable. These two negative qualities bear an obvious relation to one another and to the vulnerability of the profession to misdirected criticism. The idea of education as social repression has force simply because it reflects a great deal of historical truth. For example, in 1839 in his preface to *Nicholas Nickleby,* Dickens lashed out with the following tirade:

> Although any man who had proved his unfitness for any other occupation in life, was free, without examination or qualification, to open a school anywhere; although preparation for the functions he undertook, was required in the surgeon who assisted to bring a boy into the world, or might one day assist, perhaps, to send him out of it; in the chemist, the attorney, the butcher, the baker, the candlestick-maker; the whole round of crafts and trades, the schoolmaster excepted; and although schoolmasters, as a race, were the blockheads and imposters who might naturally be expected to spring from such a state of things, and to flourish in it; these Yorkshire schoolmasters were the lowest and most rotten round in the whole ladder. Traders in the avarice, indifference, or imbecility of parents, and the helplessness of children; ignorant, sordid, brutal men, to whom few considerate persons would have entrusted the board and lodging of a horse or a dog; they formed the worthy cornerstone of a structure, which, for absurdity and a magnificent high-minded laissez-aller neglect, has rarely been exceeded in the world.

When public dissatisfaction with educational outcomes increases, a frequent tactic is the baiting of the straw man of the teacher as a tool of repressive forces. (The most recent version of this argument allies stimulant-prescribing physicians with label-happy educators in a plot to crush individual differences; cf. "LD leaders strike back at distorted reporting," 1975.) In reality, it is striking how immune children are to the occasional teacher who is either incompetent or suffering from a personality disorder. In other words, a reasonable range of teacher variability (i.e., eccentricity) appears to have little impact on most children.

MATERIALS AND METHODS

A good teacher will teach well regardless of the theory he suffers from.

Barth
The Sot-Weed Factor

Three quarters of a century ago, Huey (1908) described the teaching of reading as "an old curiosity shop of absurd practices." Recently, Gibson and Levin (1975) could still depict the teaching of reading as faddish, with each new method being "widely trumpeted, vociferously defended, and then abandoned except by a few faithful acolytes."

When children are placed in special reading groups, an initial transient spurt is noted; but this is not maintained for longer than 6 months, and by 2 years the gains are disappointingly small (Curr and Gourlay, 1953; cf. Appendix B). This pessimistic prognosis is independent of instructional method (Silberberg, Iverson, and Goins, 1973). Phonics versus whole-word, multimodal (VAKT) versus unimodal, initial teaching alphabet (i.t.a.) versus regular orthography are all shibboleths used to disguise a basic failure (cf. Bryan and Bryan, 1975; Downing, 1973; Flesch, 1956). When a child fails with one approach, it is taken as evidence for the innate superiority of the opposite methodology, and when that approach exhibits its proportion of failures, names are changed and the cycle starts again.

Chall's (1967) conclusion that it is impossible to teach all children to read by any one method can be expanded for the learning-disabled child: 1) it is impossible to teach all learning-disabled children by any one method, 2) it may be impossible to predict which method will work best with a given specific learning disability (SLD) child, and 3) there may exist children for whom no approach is successful.

The training of specific perceptual processes has no effect on educational achievement (I. Belmont and Birch, 1974; cf. A. A. Silver, Hagin, and Hersh, 1967). To a certain extent the amount of reading improvement is related directly to the time spent teaching reading and is unrelated to the time spent on perceptual skills or language arts (Camp, 1973; A. J. Harris, 1970). On the one hand, Cashdan and Pumfrey (1969) found that multiplying the hours of remedial help by three did not accelerate reading attainment; on the other hand, Balow (1965) noted that discontinuation of remedial reading markedly decreased the rate of reading progress. Separate from actual reading achievement, Cashdan et al. (1971) could not even document a healthier and more positive attitude toward reading on the part of children who had received remedial instruction.

Recent attempts to make reading instruction more scientific have focused on aptitude-treatment interactions (ATI) as a basis for diagnostic prescriptive teaching. This approach assumes that a modality preference (identified by tests that regardless of claims to the contrary are at bottom perceptual) for processing information has definite implications for the remediation of learning disabilities. Research, however, has not supported an interaction between specific perceptual abilities or information-processing preferences and educational achievement (Newcomer and Goodman, 1975; Ringler and Smith, 1973; Sabatino and Dorfman, 1974; Sabatino, Ysseldyke, and Woolston, 1973; Waugh, 1973). The matching of instructional materials and methods to presumed auditory, visual, tactile, or kinesthetic deficits is at the least premature.

Intuitively it seems reasonable to suppose that a careful evaluation of a child's strengths and weaknesses would be useful in curriculum planning for this particular child. It has not, however, been possible to generalize this hypothesis to allow research verification (cf. Tarver and Dawson, 1978). Whether through inadequate research design, insufficiently sensitive measurement tools, or some other deficiency (e.g., invalid hypothesis), existing outcome studies do not justify a refined subgrouping of learning-disabled children; there is little evidence that different types of reading problems respond to different methods (Yule, 1976). While such classifications remain a matter of faith, it is imperative that the children not be penalized for not complying with the expectancies generated by unproved dogma. Indeed, the failure of such deficit-centered training may be considered to provide indirect support for a more global underlying problem, such as an attentional deficit (cf. Dykman et al., 1971; Rourke, 1975). The diagnostic-prescriptive model reflects a mechanistic fitting of the child to the reading program like a key to a lock (cf. Sapir and Wilson, 1978); as such it is a modern survival of Cartesian dualism. The missing perceptual/processing links used to shore up this crumbling edifice will ultimately share the fate of Piltdown man.

The nature of the classroom structure has fostered much debate. Self-contained classrooms of less than a dozen children may be needed for children with significant neurobehavioral symptoms or secondary emotional problems. Even smaller groups may be optimal for the child with a severe learning disorder. A high teacher-pupil ratio enables a greater degree of individualized instruction. The extent to which SLD children may be mainstreamed (regular class placement with resource room help in the weakest subjects) must remain the subject of trial-and-error and requires a careful, periodic monitoring of academic gains and behavioral adjustment.

Flynn and Rapoport (1976) described the *open classroom* with clear, explicit guidelines, in which the teacher can deal with conflicts and disruptive behavior without involving the group and in which the emotional climate is warm and accepting, as the *preferred* environment for hyperactive children. Other studies of the open classroom have not been as positive. In the areas of academic achievement, creativity, and social and emotional adjustment, the formal or traditional classroom was equal to or better than the open classroom (Bennett, 1976; Ward and Barcher, 1975). Open and nongraded classrooms are excellent in theory but are often misunderstood and misused in practice (Sapir and Wilson, 1978). Like many other methodologies that do exceptionally well in experimental situations, they are nowhere near as effective in general practice because they assume an exceptionally zealous, expert, and creative teacher when the available teacher is one of average training and ability (A. J. Harris, 1970). Mainstreaming and the open classroom do not necessarily represent the "least restrictive environment" for the SLD child; indeed, for such children they may be extremely restricting (Cruickshank, 1977). Bureaucratically, administratively, and financially, such options, with their deemphasis of diagnosis (Foster, Schmidt, and Sabatino, 1976), have much to offer all concerned, except the children.

THE TEACHER

Unfortunately teachers, although they claim to be members of a profession, do not enjoy the authority to the same degree of a credentialed group, as do engineers, physicians, and lawyers.

Broudy (1976)

At present there is no educational technology guaranteed to prevent or cure specific learning disabilities. The optimal program for teachers to follow is the one best suited to their personal abilities and training and adapted to the individual pupil's needs (cf. A. J. Harris, 1970; Harris and Sipay, 1975) as determined by a trial of teaching rather than psychoeducational test scores. This is similar to the situation where a needed surgical procedure can be performed by a variety of different operations with only minimal differences with regard to mortality, morbidity, and outcome; the critical variable becomes the individual surgeon's training and experience.

Chall (1967) observed that the teacher was the most important element in a reading program. It should not be a matter of great surprise that the crucial characteristics in the management of SLD children turn out to be human traits rather than mechanistic variables. Thus the following comments: "Skilled and sympathetic individual teaching, without application of undue pressure and with frequent reinforcement by praise and reassurance, is at present the optimal management" (Kinsbourne, 1968); any remedial approach that includes individual attention, sympathetic understanding, and parental involvement will help (Bettman et al., 1967). Such approaches will not necessarily accelerate academic achievement but will perhaps prevent the incidence of secondary behavioral manifestations.

As to describing the ideal learning disabilities teacher, John Baptist de la Salle's (1651–1719) 12 virtues of a good teacher remain the best approximation: wisdom, prudence, piety, zeal, generosity, justice, kindness, firmness, humility, patience, seriousness, and silence (Grande, 1962). A healthy degree of skepticism with regard to methodology and a sense of humor are all that is needed to complete this profile. Education, like medicine, is severely limited in its ability to screen persons with the appropriate academic and intellectual credentials, in order to determine their adequacy as human beings. In 1951, Barnes predicted that "some day we shall have a science of education comparable to the science of medicine; but even when that day arrives the *art* of education will still remain the inspiration and the guide of all wise teachers." The art of the wise teacher seems to be identical to the art of being human.

ACCOUNTABILITY

What is there that a doctor can usefully say to a teacher?

D. W. Winnicott
The Child, The Family, and the Outside World

Prevailing concepts of educational accountability are open to criticism: "In most jobs, if a man does not do what he is paid to do, he is considered a failure. In teaching, when that happens, the *student* is considered a failure" (Postman and Weingartner, 1971). While malpractice suits (or their equivalent) have long exerted an influence on medical practice, it has only been in the past decade that attempts have been made to recover compensation for educational incompetence. Dickens *(Nicholas Nickleby)* had suggested the analogy:

> We hear sometimes of an action for damages against the unqualified medical practitioner, who has deformed a broken limb in pretending to heal it. But, what of the hundreds thousands of minds that have been deformed for ever by the incapable pettifoggers who have pretended to form them!

The weeding out of gross incompetence and personality disorders is in the province of the profession, but education, like medicine, has difficulties measuring and rewarding competence and performance above minimal standards.

The Education for All Handicapped Children Act (PL 94-142) now requires the school system to develop an individualized education program (IEP) for each child receiving special services; this IEP must, at least annually, include in writing the following:

1. Current level of functioning
2. Short- and long-term goals
3. Type and duration of special intervention to be provided
4. Evaluation criteria that will be used to determine whether the projected goals have been met on schedule

The precise implications of the IEP for teacher accountability remain unclear, but there does appear to be some risk that in order to guarantee success, the goals may be kept minimal (cf. Sapir and Wilson, 1978). This will be in striking contrast to the overly optimistic predictions that are almost traditional for SLD children. The most reasonable solution to this dilemma is a multidisciplinary approach, with a team evaluation by a pediatrician with expertise in developmental disabilities, a skilled child psychologist, and a special educator; the first two should preferably come from outside the school, the third will supervise the provision of services and help to continuously monitor their efficacy from within the system.

It has been claimed that the medical evaluation is irrelevant to the remediation of learning problems. The difficulty with this charge is that the medical model is only a specific application of the scientific model (cf. Kauffman and Hallahan, 1974). Human variables, which make measurement and modification difficult, do prevent the classroom from mirroring laboratory results. Medicine offers no specifics on teaching strategies and methods except to reinforce a critical skepticism of an overreliance on unproved (if not disproved) technologies, a criticism whose proper source is education itself. The physician can also help the educator to establish a valid framework for estimating the magnitude of educational gains to be expected and to more realistically evaluate program effectiveness (Reed, 1979). The medical examination that in itself does not alter the outcome for SLD children may yet help to explain why educational intervention has little effect on outcome for a certain group of children. Any model that focuses too exclusively on changing the child risks failing to give adequate weight to the alternatives that it may be school, parental, and societal expectations that need to be changed and that "changed" is not equivalent to "lowered." The pediatrician is the advocate for these alternatives.

OUTCOME

Most studies of younger minimal brain dysfunction (MBD)/SLD children suggest that the disorder will respond either to time or to appropriate intervention so that by adolescence and adulthood these children will be grossly indistinguishable from their peers.

Laufer (1971) found that 70% of his patients were later either in college or gainfully employed. But while the basic underlying disorder may improve and its manifestations change, favorable long-term outcomes appear to be questionable.

All the following studies report group results that suggest that, independent of intelligence and social class, MBD/SLD children do significantly worse than their peers in adult educational attainment and degree of social adjustment. The averaged percentages conceal the fact that a number of these children do considerably worse (and considerably better) than these lowered means. Again, some of the studies refer to learning-disabled children, others to reading disorders, several to dyslexia, and a number to minimal brain dysfunction or hyperkinesis. Some of them control for IQ, socioeconomic status (SES), and other variables; others do not. Only a few utilize a group of matched controls. Despite the use of equivalent definitions of the initial diagnosis, biases in the nature of the children referred to different research centers make interstudy comparisons even more difficult. Finally, a difference of 10 or more years in the length of the follow-up or in the date of the study might question the relevance of research findings to current practices. Despite all these qualifications and its own inconsistencies, the literature is fairly unanimous: the prognosis for MBD/SLD children is not good.

M. Menkes, Rowe, and Menkes (1967) reported a persistence of hyperactivity in 20% of MBD subjects after 25 years; at follow-up 20% had criminal records and almost a third were suffering from psychoses. More striking, there was no apparent correlation between later social adjustment and either early home environment or the amount of therapeutic intervention. Half of hyperactive children between 12 and 16 years of age had markedly improved, but most were still troubled by symptoms and almost two-thirds had had some trouble with the law (Mendelson, Johnson, and Stewart, 1971). Ackerman, Dykman, and Peters (1977b) found that half of their MBD/SLD adolescents had major conflicts with authority and a third demonstrated psychological disturbances; Laufer (1971) noted a lower rate (30%) of trouble with the law. Huessy, Metoyer, and Townsend (1974) reported that institutionalization for delinquency or psychiatric reasons was 20 times higher than normal in hyperkinetic children at follow-up in adolescence and could find no correlation between outcome and drug therapy, drug responsiveness, or duration of treatment.

Weiss et al. (1971, 1975; Minde, Weiss, and Mendelson, 1972) concluded that long-term methylphenidate had no statistically significant impact on later emotional adjustment, delinquency, or academic performance.

It is estimated that somewhere between 25% and 75% of all juvenile delinquency is related to organic brain dysfunction, with the typical adolescent delinquent being 3 to 5 years delayed in academic skills, and reading being more retarded than mathematics (Poremba, 1975). Again, Margolin, Roman, and Harari (1955) found that 75% of juvenile delinquents were 2 years behind in reading and more than 50% were 5 or more years behind. Cantwell (1972, 1978; cf. Hechtman et al., 1976; Minde et al., 1971) had noted an increased incidence of delinquency and antisocial behavior in MBD children. In an evaluation of adolescents who had attempted suicide, 60% had histories and assessments consistent with earlier MBD, and 75% had exceptionally poor school records (Rohn et al., 1977). A probably related finding is the higher rate of occurrence of automobile accidents involving persons who had been hyperactive children (Hechtman et al., 1976).

Long-term educational outcomes for MBD/SLD children are the subject of conflicting reports. In a dyslexic population with a mean IQ of 91.8, Rabinovitch et al. (1956) noted persistent difficulties in reading as opposed to Rawson's (1968) more optimistic findings in a group of "dyslexic" children with a mean IQ of 130.8. More than half of a group of reading-disordered children with a mean IQ of 120 completed college (H. M. Robinson and Smith, 1962). Similarly, Weiss et al. (1971) noted that MBD children with higher IQs were succeeding in school.

Balow and Blomquist (1965) surveyed reading-disabled children 10 to 15 years after their initial evaluation and found an average adult reading grade level of 10; although these children surpassed their fathers in educational achievement, they held lower-level jobs (cf. P. T. Rogers et al., in preparation). In Borland and Heckman's (1976) study, the level of education achieved was lower for hyperkinetic males than for their brothers. Tarnopol (1969c) reported that 58% of learning-disabled children were below a sixth grade reading level as adults; Franuenheim (1978) noted that despite special educational intervention, the average adult reading level for dyslexic children was 3.6 years. Finally, the school dropout rate for hyperkinetic children is 5 times higher than in the general population (Huessy et al., 1974).

In general, most reading-disabled children become literate, but few read at an average level (Muehl and Forell, 1973). Persistent deficiencies on psychological and perceptual tasks seem related to the care with which such deficits are searched for (Ackerman, Dykman, and Peters, 1977a; Silver and Hagin, 1964). Those learning-disabled children with the more severe early reading problems seem to have the poorest later outcomes (Ackerman, et al., 1977a); otherwise, the level of hyperkinesis, family history, and the presence of neurological signs all appear unrelated to eventual academic achievement. No special intervention—medical, educational, or psychological—radically alters the outcome.

Again, it must be emphasized that this "poor" outcome is a statistical phenomenon; individual MBD/SLD children will do better or worse than the group mean. The critical problem facing professionals working with such children is a total incapability of identifying the variables (either diagnostic or therapeutic) that will improve outcomes for particular children. The descriptive classification MBD/SLD then becomes a restatement of the observation that the child with a learning disorder is "at risk" to do poorly (i.e., not as well as might be predicted from IQ and SES) in later life. The extent to which time or remediation will affect the ultimate outcome cannot be predicted, given the current state of knowledge.

CONCLUSION
AND SUMMARY

It's a failure of national vision when you regard children as weapons, and talents as materials you can mine, assay, and fabricate for profit and defense.

John Hersey
The Child Buyer

The ancients placed the vital center sometimes in the heart, sometimes in the liver; moderns are unanimous in locating it in the brain. Having centered human nature in the brain, human worth is frequently identified with cognitive measures, such as level of academic attainment and all its correlates. Szasz (1974) has warned of the dangers to human liberty of such a reductionist perspective: "The more man's view of human nature emphasizes material values, scientific determinism, and human equality and perfectibility, the greater will be the scope of controlling conduct through external coercion." It is difficult if not impossible for schools to escape the prevalent value system; some consolation can be found in the fact that schools do not always succeed in producing children according to the advertised model (cf. Skidelsky, 1970).

Perceptual theories (and all their disguised variants) of learning disability are similar to schools of philosophy and theology: each age sees arrogant youth dragging the corpses of their predecessors around the arena (Mottram, 1952). At bottom, perception is more than just a stage in cognitive development; it is one of the languages into which prelinquistic thought (Chomsky's deep structure) is translated. Although the experimental evidence is not complete, perceptual, sequencing, and memory skills; gross motor output; and fine motor coordination are all significantly related to verbal fluency (cf. Bryan and Bryan, 1975; Luria, 1961; Wolff and Wolff, 1972). If there exists a single (and by no means least) common denominator to the variegated symptomatology of the minimal brain dysfunction (MBD)/specific learning disorder (SLD) complex, it is linguistic in nature.

The claim that the management of learning disabilities is the exclusive province of the educator is untenable; it makes the absurd assumption that all significant learning takes place in the school. (Alternatively, teaching failure in the school setting has been used to argue for a more pervasive role for education with intervention in the home and preschool environments.) Schooling does have a profound effect on cognitive skills, but it will never succeed in equalizing them (Jencks et al., 1972; Stevenson et al., 1978). As long as that uniformity of outcome remains a goal, schools (i.e., their expectations, not their tests) will generate failure and suffering. The assumption that more expensive technologies are required where the less costly ones have failed is false; what is really needed is a change in attitude—not a lowering of expectations (although by formal testing, this may be the case) but a readjustment of priorities, a certain flexibility and willingness of the system to bend. SLD children can learn, but not with prepackaged remedial programs; the cant of individualized teaching needs to be replaced by the reality. Less can sometimes be more effective than more, especially if the less is tolerant, considerate and caring, and child-centered rather than curriculum-centered.

Even with our present confused state of knowledge, teachers would benefit greatly in their training from an increased exposure to course material on the organic substrates of learning; as it is, they generally receive a very one-sided psychosocial orientation (cf. Reed, 1979). Soon, educators whose focus is narrowed exclusively to sociocultural determinants will with little preparation find themselves contending with direct biological manipulations of learning ability (cf. McGaugh, 1976). Although educational studies to date are rather pessimistic, the concept of organic, neurologically based limitations (i.e., innate or relatively fixed individual differences) is not necessarily therapeutically nihilistic; at the least the behavioral and social outcomes should be amenable to change. An older wisdom reminds us that it should not be necessary to hope in order to undertake nor to succeed in order to persevere.

SUMMARY

In my end is my beginning.

T. S. Eliot, "East Coker"

What the physician diagnoses as minimal brain dysfunction is what the educator labels specific learning disability; both of these terms encompass an indeterminant number of heterogeneous subgroups with different presentations and prognoses.

There is no generally accepted subclassification scheme of proved utility.

The importance of the term *MBD* lies in its focus on an organic contribution to disorders of learning and behavior in childhood; employment of more specific labels or no diagnostic term at all (but rather process-oriented descriptions of children's learning behavior) have generated a great deal of enthusiasm but little scientific support.

The most important component of the MBD syndrome is not hyperactivity but an SLD; organic hyperactivity derives from the pervasiveness of the learning disability.

Minimal diagnostic criteria for the MBD/SLD complex have not been defined; although a pediatrician, psychologist, or teacher may suspect this syndrome, no one of these specialists can confirm the diagnosis without input from the other two.

Emotional disturbance as a cause of MBD/SLD is extremely rare; secondary emotional disturbances, on the other hand, are very common. Before psychiatric referral, the appropriateness of the class placement should be determined and, if necessary, corrected.

Although learning disabilities cannot be screened accurately in the preschool population, the most sensitive indicator for later learning problems is the presence of an early language disorder (i.e., delayed onset of speech, delay or deviancy in language milestones, disarticulation).

The long-term outlook for MBD/SLD is neither optimistic nor pessimistic, but rather guarded; problems with learning and behavior can persist in modified form into adulthood (i.e., learning-disabled children do not necessarily catch up or grow out of their problem by adolescence).

All new diagnostic tools and therapeutic modalities should be greeted with a skepticism directly proportional to the popular enthusiasm they generate.

Medical, psychological, and educational evaluation and treatment have not been documented to have any long-term effect on outcome for MBD/SLD children. In view of this, a great deal of prudence is required in order to delineate the extent of the evaluation and the nature of the treatment.

Dietary manipulation works for an extremely small subgroup of the MBD/SLD population, but it is nowhere near as effective as psychostimulants. Its almost paranoid faddishness contributes to an increasing medicalization of daily life (i.e., food as drug or toxin).

Optometric exercises and other forms of vision therapy have no place in the treatment of learning disability.

Occupational therapy has no proved role in the evaluation and treatment of learning disability.

Dyscalculia and dysgraphia represent uncharted territories.

Handedness, especially as related to mixed dominance, is a red herring.

The pediatrician is by training and logistically the professional of choice to provide ongoing family counseling and multidisciplinary team management. Failure to maintain adequate communication with the child's teacher is the pediatrician's greatest weakness.

Psychostimulants, appropriately monitored, can enhance attentional ability, self-control, and independence.

Perinatal complications and certain infant behavior patterns are associated with later disorders of learning and behavior in children; however, this relationship is not clinically predictive.

Soft neurological signs and minor malformations are associated with both MBD/SLD and mental retardation, but this correlation is not diagnostic.

Computerized electroencephalographic (EEG) interpretations may statistically distinguish drug responses, but routine EEGs have no place in the evaluation of MBD/SLD children.

Perceptual-motor tests are so unreliable that they cannot accurately discriminate learning disabilities and should not be used to measure academic progress.

Routine use of projective tests in MBD/SLD children is unwarranted.

Problems with social learning are often ignored relative to the stress placed on academic achievement.

There is no one IQ score for any child.

Significant subscore scatter may occur independent of significant verbal-performance IQ differences (and vice versa).

Significant verbal-performance IQ differences and/or subscore scatter may occur in the absence of a learning disability.

A child with a learning disability may demonstrate neither a verbal-performance IQ discrepancy nor subscore scatter.

MBD/SLD learning patterns occur in children with more significant brain damage (e.g., mental retardation and cerebral palsy) with high frequency. (The brain damage model provides one of the most effective paradigms for understanding the MBD/SLD child.)

Behavior psychology (learning theory) can offer a useful adjunct for both the physician and the teacher in their approach to the MBD/SLD child.

Sensory modality preference approaches (e.g., Illinois Test of Psycholinguistic Abilities, diagnostic-prescriptive teaching) have not demonstrated any significant impact on learning-disabled children.

No single reading/teaching method can be employed successfully with all children; no single remedial approach is effective with all learning-disabled children.

The efficacy of any and all forms of educational intervention remains unproved; preliminary data actually render it suspect.

The most significant variable in special education is the teacher, but the special characteristics that define her effectiveness are unknown (i.e., teaching is an art).

From a design point of view, the majority of educational tests are poorly constructed; compared with the subjectivity in the pediatric evaluation and the variance in the psychological assessment, the accuracy of the educational profile exhibits the greatest dependency on the tact, skill, and experience of the individual examiner.

The most effective interdisciplinary team is the smallest (e.g., pediatrician, psychologist, child's teacher, and parents).

The problem of the MBD/SLD child reflects a broad philosophical issue—societal acceptance of (organic and limiting but not unworkable) individual differences.

APPENDIX A:
Reading Grade Levels

In the evaluation of a child's reading level, use is made either of a series of graded readers or graded reading passages (informal assessment) or of a standardized reading test (formal assessment). Occasionally the readability level of material outside such sources is desired. For the physician involved in human research or research review, the grade levels of consent forms (especially child assent forms) may need to be estimated. Two commonly used measures require the same input data: average sentence length (SL) and average word length in syllables (WL). These are calculated for random 100-word samples at the beginning, middle, and end of

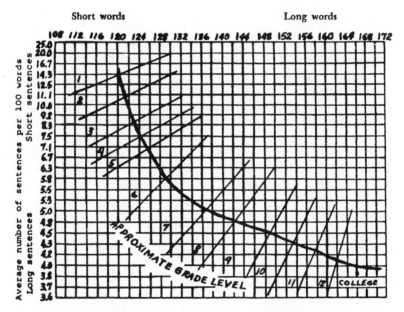

DIRECTIONS: Randomly select 3 one hundred word passages from a book or an article. Plot average number of syllables and average number of words per sentence on graph to determine area of readability level. Choose more passages per book if great variability is observed.

Figure A.1. Fry graph for estimating readability. (From E. Fry, 1968.)

Table A.1.   Reading grade levels for common materials

Author	Work	Reading grade level Flesch	Fry
Baum	*Wizard of Oz*	6.7	7
Milne	*Winnie the Pooh*	7.2	7
Dickens	*A Christmas Carol*	7.5	7
Ruskin	*King of the Golden River*	7.8	7
IRS	"1978 Tax Instructions"	8.9	9
Tolstoy	*War and Peace*	9.7	11
New York Times	Editorial page	10.5	12

the work. Grade level may then be predicted by Flesch's (1948) formula:

$$C_{75} = 0.0846WL + 0.1015SL - 5.6835$$

where C_{75} is the average grade of children who could answer 75% of the test questions correctly, or by plotting WL and SL on the Fry graph (Figure A.1). These two methods are compared in Table A.1. An alternative procedure, the Harris-Jacobson Readability Formulas (A. J. Harris and Sipay, 1975; Appendix B), involves comparison with standard word lists.

Average word length is an indirect measure of word complexity, and average sentence length is an indirect measure of sentence complexity and abstraction. However, short words and short sentences do not always make for simplicity; a passage composed of short sentences on the order of abstraction of "to be or not to be" would yield an erroneously low reading grade level. Botel and Granowsky (1972) have proposed a preliminary scale to quantitatively measure syntactical complexity.

APPENDIX B:
Rate of Reading Achievement

Reading achievement is similar to intelligence in that predictability is lower and variability is greater as one progresses toward the bright end of the spectrum. In normal children, reading progress is so variable it is described as idiosyncratic (I. Belmont and Belmont, 1978). Although reading progress in the severely learning disabled, like intelligence in the more severely retarded, may be more predictable, there is no single generally accepted measure of progress in reading. This makes the assessment of research papers and intervention programs as well as the counseling of individual students difficult. As will be seen, the reason for this absence of a standard for comparison is simply that all of the instruments designed for this purpose are seriously flawed. Clinicians and researchers ought not to select a method that fits their preconceptions without first realizing its limitations.

One of the simplest measures of reading progress is the reading quotient (RQ), in which reading age (RA) is divided by chronological age (CA):

$$RQ = RA/CA \times 100$$

Both the numerator and denominator can be converted to grade levels rather than age levels by subtracting 5.2, since 6.2 years is the average age of starting first grade. Grade ratios and age ratios yield identical results for the child performing up to expectancy, but they will diverge more markedly as reading performance declines compared to chronological age. Most reading tests introduce the additional artifact of starting a child at a beginning first grade level (1.0); this represents a baseline of 6.2 years in both the numerator and denominator of an age ratio and will obscure delays for the first several years of school. The age ratio will, however, more accurately reflect reading progress at an earlier grade level than the grade ratio (Figure B.1). In comparison, by the third to fourth grade, the correlation between reading and IQ becomes substantial (Bloom, 1964; A. J. Harris, 1970).

Monroe (1932) proposed the following reading index (RI):

$$RI = \frac{RA}{(MA + CA + \text{Arithmetic age})/3}$$

All the age levels are actually expressed in grade levels, and the reading age is the average of four separate reading test scores. The mean RI is 1.0, with a standard deviation of 0.2; an $RI < 0.8$ is considered significant. A. J. Harris (1970) simplified Monroe's for-

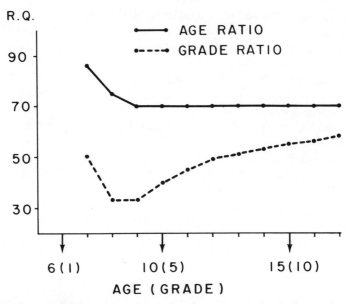

Figure B.1. Reading quotient. In the first few years of school, the use of reading tests to form a reading quotient (RQ), whether by an age ratio or a grade ratio, can be highly misleading. The figure plots hypothetical RQs for a child whose reading and language abilities have been progressing at a constant 70% of normal; the artifactual acceleration and decelerations are caused by the use of a reading test with a basal score of 1.0.

mula by transferring the weight given to arithmetic to mental age:

$$\text{Reading expectancy age (REA)}= \frac{2MA+CA}{3}$$

$$\text{Reading expectancy quotient (REQ)}=\frac{RA}{REA}\times 100$$

As the child's arithmetic achievement age moves closer to his mental age than to his reading age, the RI and the REA approximate each other. An REQ < 90 is considered significantly low, whereas an REQ > 110 reflects overachievement. A. J. Harris and Sipay (1975) use both the REQ and the simpler RQ to profile reading-delayed children.

Bond and Tinker (1973) suggested that expected reading grade level was best predicted by:

$$(\text{Years in school}\times \frac{IQ}{100})+1 \text{ year}=\text{Expected reading grade}$$

By weighting experience (years in school), this formula would better compensate for the clinical impression that low-IQ children tend to overachieve and high-IQ children tend to underachieve when compared with predictions based solely on intelligence and/or chronological age. In a variation on this formula, Myklebust (1968, 1973) offered a calculation for expectancy age:

$$\text{Expectancy age} = \frac{MA + CA + \text{Grade age}}{3}$$

The learning quotient derived from this formula is significantly low if it is below 90. A comparison of some of these formulas to mental age predictions is presented in Figure B.2. For the child who: 1) has an IQ of 100, 2) is in an age-appropriate grade, and 3) is doing grade-appropriate work, all these reading quotients produce scores of 100. For the child who is underachieving, those formulas that yield quotients further from 100 on initial assessment will magnify any change that occurs on reevaluation.

Population studies have yielded several sets of multiple regression equations that predict reading age from chronological age and verbal IQ (Figure B.3). The standard errors for the reading levels produced by these equations (i.e., by these population studies) approach 2 years; when these reading levels are converted into reading quotients, these standard errors can account for differences on the magnitude of 20 points. Despite the possibility of significant differences between the standardization sample for a specific reading test and the local clinical population, such large standard errors make it unlikely that regional norms will ever be of much help to the individual child performing near the lower end of the distribution (cf. Silberberg, Iversen, and Silberberg, 1969). When the curves derived from population studies are superimposed on several of those predictive indices described earlier, it appears that throughout elementary school mental age is a better predictor of reading age than the more complex formulae (Figure B.4).

Another instrument to compare reading achievement with intelligence is the Z-score discrepancy method (Erickson, 1975; Muzyczka and Erickson, 1976; Savage, 1968). Both the IQ and the reading score are transformed into Z-scores (the number of standard deviations from the mean for each test for each score, respectively) and the two Z-scores are compared. (A variation on this procedure is employed in Savage and O'Connor, 1966). While

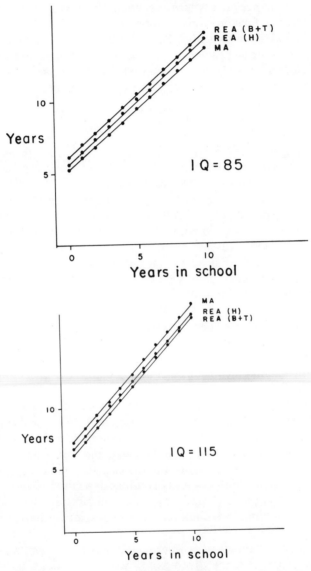

Figure B.2. Reading expectancy level. If reading were perfectly correlated with intelligence, then the reading expectancy level for bright and dull children would be expected to match their mental age (MA). Several formulas have tried to take into account the facts that bright children underachieve and dull children over-achieve: Reading expectancy age=2MA+Chronological age)/3 (A. J. Harris, 1970); Reading expectancy grade=(Years in school × IQ/100)+1 (Bond and Tinker, 1973); Reading age=Reading grade+5.2 (A. J. Harris, 1970).

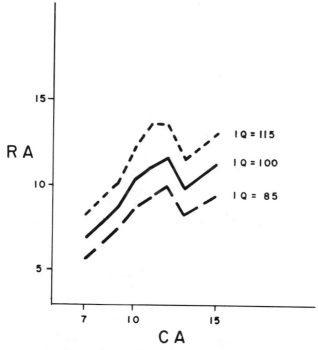

Figure B.3. Reading age from chronological age and verbal IQ. The curves for three different verbal IQs were plotted from Fransella and Gerver's (1966) multiple regression equations: ages 6–9: $RA = -8.44 + (0.98 \times CA) + (0.085 \times IQ)$; ages 10–12: $RA = -7.68 + (0.64 \times CA) + (0.117 \times IQ)$; ages 13–15: $RA = -10.86 + (0.72 \times CA) + (0.144 \times IQ)$. Similar formulas have been derived from population studies by Savage and O'Connor (1966) and Yule (1967).

other formulas overidentify low-IQ children as reading underachievers, the Z-score method identifies a higher proportion of normal- to high-IQ children as reading disabled. This method is predominantly for use in identification; there are no data on its use to follow rate of reading progress (e.g., stability of Z-score discrepancy over time).

Two simpler methods of assessing reading progress are the years below method (cf. Erickson, 1975) and the annual rate method. The years below method records how many years or months a child's reading level is behind his actual grade placement; it does not usually allow for intelligence level or whether the grade placement is appropriate for age (e.g., whether the child has been left back). Furthermore, there is no consideration given to

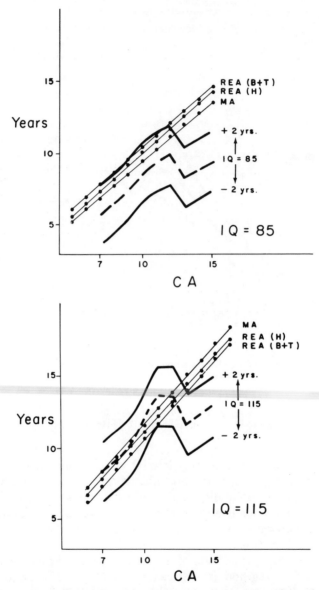

Figure B.4. Fransella and Gerver's (1966) regression equations for each of two IQ levels are superimposed on the reading expectancy levels described previously. It appears that throughout most of elementary school the population described by the regression equations approximates mental age (MA) expectations more closely than do the other two formulas. (The curves above and below the dashed regression equation curves indicate the standard error of ± 2 grade levels.)

the fact that many severely learning disabled children will *at best* fall further behind academically over time. To say that a half-grade behind is acceptable in the first half of grade school and a full grade behind is acceptable in the second half does not begin to respond to the needs of individual students for whom such cutoffs may be gross over- or underestimates.

The annual rate method forms the ratio (months of progress in reading)/10 months and monitors changes in this ratio each school year. This method is probably most useful when combined with one of the other reading quotients discussed; alone, it can be very misleading. A typical learning-disabled child may demonstrate poor reading progress over the first 2 to 3 years of school; placed in a special reading class, he then shows marked improvement over the next year. His second year in the special class produces little further improvement (indeed, with the annual rate method he may have a negative progress score for this year), and he is judged ready to be returned to the regular class. In reality his reading performance in the first few years of school represented a relative underachievement secondary to inappropriate class placement; his dramatic improvement during his first year in the special class reflected a number of factors, including a closer approximation to his potential in an optimal educational environment and a degree of regression toward the mean. The marked acceleration in such classes rarely survives the first year; by the end of the second year there is a plateau effect that is frequently misinterpreted as implying that this particular child has gotten all that he can from such special placement. He may actually need this special class continued in order to maintain his expectedly slow rate of progress. Special (reading) classes may occasionally produce miracles, but that is not their purpose; they are there to serve the children for whom there are no miracles.

BIBLIOGRAPHICAL
NOTE

Let me recommend this book—one of the most re-
markable ever penned.

Conan Doyle
The Sign of the Four

Capute and Accardo (1980), Kinsbourne and Caplan (1979), and
Peters et al. (1973) are general introductions to the MBD/SLD
spectrum. Several excellent anthologies on the process of reading
are Kavanagh and Mattingly (1972), LaBerge and Samuels (1977),
and Levin and Williams (1970). Downing's (1973) work on comparative reading is a gold mine of data. Huey's (1908) classic text
is still well worth reading, and Gibson and Levin's (1975) review of
the psychology of reading is magisterial. From an educational
standpoint, see Bond and Tinker (1973), A. J. Harris (1970), A. J.
Harris and Sipay (1975), and De Cecco (1968). The language background is covered in Rutter and Martin (1972). Hyperactivity is
reviewed exhaustively in Safer and Allen (1976) and Ross and
Ross (1976).

Much of the discussion of the Wechsler Intelligence Scale for
Children (WISC) in this book is derived directly or indirectly from
Sattler (1974). The pediatric member of the interdisciplinary team
should observe the test being given several times, he should
review the manual (Wechsler, 1974), and he should familiarize
himself with A. S. Kaufman's two papers (1976a, b). Neuropsychology is reviewed in Knights and Bakker (1976) and Reitan and
Davison (1974). More traditional approaches to the psychological
assessment of children are found in Allen and Allen (1967), Anastasi (1968), Cronbach (1970), and Taylor (1961). The problems
associated with the use of psychological tests on minority children are discussed in Oakland (1977) and Wright and Isenstein
(1977). Suggestions for constructing an office assessment battery
are made by Desmond et al. (1978), Hartlage and Lucas (1973),
Klapper (1966), and Peters et al. (1973). Specific psychoeducational tests are critically reviewed in Buros (1972, 1974), Mauser
(1977), and Sapir and Wilson (1978).

Paine and Oppé (1966) remains the best introduction to the
pediatric neurological examination; a profusion of test forms can
be found in *Pharmacotherapy of Children* (1973). Several works
provide useful introductions to relevant areas of neuroanatomy
and neurophysiology: Luria (1961, 1963, 1973), Magoun (1963),

and Mountcastle (1962). The rationale for and clinical experience with psychostimulants are reviewed in books by Conners (1974b), Kinsbourne and Caplan (1979, especially Chapter 9), White (1977), and J. M. Wiener (1977, especially the chapters by Conners and Cantwell) and papers, by Barkley (1977), Forman (1975), Whalen and Henker (1976), and Wolraich (1977). The biochemical background is presented in D. J. Cohen and Young (1977) and S. E. Shaywitz et al. (1978), with neurotransmitter physiology being reviewed in Axelrod (1974) and Pincus and Tucker (1974).

Principles of behavior management (for parents, teachers, and physicians) are presented in Becker (1971), Deibert and Harman (1973), Krumboltz and Krumboltz (1972), Madsen and Madsen (1974), Patterson (1975), Patterson and Gullion (1971), and Werry and Wollersheim (1967). Educational professionalism is reviewed in Clifford (1975, Chapter 6).

BIBLIOGRAPHY

Aarskog, D., Fevang, F. Ø., Kløve, H., Støa, K. F., and Thorsen, T. 1977. The effect of the stimulant drugs, dextroamphetamine and methylphenidate, on secretion of growth hormone in hyperactive children. J. Pediatr. 90:136–139.

Abercrombie, M. L. J. 1968. Some notes on spatial disability: Movement, intelligence quotient and attentiveness. Dev. Med. Child Neurol. 10:206–213.

Abercrombie, M. L. J. 1970. Learning to draw. In K. Connolly (ed.), Mechanisms of Motor Skills, pp. 307–325. Academic Press, New York.

Abercrombie, M. L. J., Lindon, R. L., and Tyson, M. C. 1964. Associated movements in normal and physically handicapped children. Dev. Med. Child Neurol. 6:573–580.

Accardo, P. J., and Capute, A. J. 1979. The Pediatrician and the Developmentally Delayed Child: A Clinical Textbook on Mental Retardation. University Park Press, Baltimore.

Ackerman, P. T., Dykman, R. A., and Peters, J. E. 1977a. Learning-disabled boys as adolescents: Cognitive factors and achievement. J. Am. Acad. Child Psychiatry 16:296–313.

Ackerman, P. T., Dykman, R. A., and Peters, J. A. 1977b. Teenage status of hyperactive learning disabled boys. Am. J. Orthopsychiatry 47:577–596.

Ackerman, P. T., Peters, J. E., and Dykman, R. A. 1971. Children with specific learning disabilities: WISC profiles. J. Learn. Disabil. 4:150–166.

Adams, R. M., Kocsis, J. J., and Estes, R. E. 1974. Soft neurological signs in learning-disabled children and controls. Am. J. Dis. Child. 128:614–618.

Adamson, W. C., and Adamson, K. K. (eds.). 1979. A Handbook for Specific Learning Disabilities. Gardner Press, New York.

Ad Hoc Committee of the American Academy of Pediatrics, American Academy of Ophthalmology and Otolaryngology, and the American Association of Ophthalmology. 1972. The eye and learning disabilities. Am. Acad. Pediatr. Newsletter, January 1 (suppl.); Pediatr. News, February, pp. 65–66; Pediatrics 49:454–455.

Admissions Testing Program. 1978. Services for Handicapped Students. Educational Testing Service/College Entrance Examination Board, Princeton, N.J.

Aird, R. B., and Yamamoto, T. 1966. Behavior disorders of childhood. Electroencephalogr. Clin. Neurophysiol. 21:148–156.

Alberman, E. 1973. The early prediction of learning disorders. Dev. Med. Child Neurol. 15:202-204.

Allen, R. M., and Allen, S. P. 1967. Intellectual Evaluation of the Mentally Retarded Child: A Handbook. Western Psychological Services, Los Angeles.

Allmond, B. W. 1974. Psychological testing of children. Pediatr. Clin. North Am. 21:187-194.

AMA Council on Drugs. 1971. AMA Drug Evalautions. American Medical Association, Chicago.

Ames, L. B. 1968a. Learning disabilities: The developmental point of view. In H. R. Myklebust (ed.), Progress in Learning Disabilities, Vol. 1, pp. 39-74. Grune & Stratton, New York.

Ames, L. B. 1968b. A low intelligence quotient often not recognized as the chief cause of many learning difficulties. J. Learn. Disabil. 1:45-48.

Anastasi, A. 1968. Psychological Testing. Macmillan Publishing Co., New York.

Anderson, J. A. 1977. Neural models with cognitive implications. In D. La Berge and S. J. Samuels (eds.), Basic Processes in Reading, pp. 27-90. Lawrence Erlbaum Associates, Hillsdale, N.J.

Anderson, U. M. 1967. The incidence and significance of high frequency deafness in children. Am. J. Dis. Child. 113:560-565.

Arnold, L. E., Strobl, D., and Weisenberg, A. 1972. Hyperkinetic adult: Study of the "paradoxical" amphetamine response. JAMA 222:693-694.

Arnold, L. E., and Wender, P. H. 1974. Levoamphetamine's changing place in the treatment of children with behavior disorders. In C. K. Conners (ed.), Clinical Use of Stimulant Drugs in Children, pp. 179-191. Excerpta Medica, Amsterdam.

Arnold, L. G., and Knopp, W. 1973. The making of a myth. JAMA 223:1273-1274.

Axelrod, J. 1974. Neurotransmitters. Sci. Am. 230(6):58-71.

Axelrod, J., Mueller, R. A., Henry, J. P., and Stephens, P. M. 1970. Changes in enzymes involved in the biosynthesis and metabolism of noradrenaline and adrenaline after psychosocial stimulation. Nature 225:1059-1060.

Ayllon, T., Layman, D., and Kandel, H. J. 1975. A behavioral-educational alternative to drug control of hyperactive children. J. Appl. Behav. Anal. 8:137-146.

Ayres, A. J. 1966. Interrelation of perception, function, and treatment. J. Am. Phys. Ther. Assoc. 46:741-744.

Ayres, A. J. 1971. Characteristics of types of sensory integrative dysfunction. Am. J. Occup. Ther. 25:329–334.

Ayres, A. J. 1972a. Improving academic scores through sensory integration. J. Learn. Disabil. 5:338–343.

Ayres, A. J. 1972b. Types of sensory integrative dysfunction among disabled learners. Am. J. Occup. Ther. 26:13–18.

Ayres, A. J. 1973. Sensory Integration and Learning Disorders. Western Psychological Services, Los Angeles.

Ayres, A. J. 1977. Dichotic listening performance in learning-disabled children. Am. J. Occup. Ther. 31:441–446.

Ayres, A. J. 1978. Learning disabilities and the vestibular system. J. Learn. Disabil. 2:18–29.

Bailey, P., and David, E. W. 1942. The syndrome of obstinate progression in the cat. Proc. Soc. Exp. Biol. 51:307.

Baker, H., and Kellogg, R. 1967. A developmental study of children's scribblings. Pediatrics 40:382–389.

Bakwin, H. 1973. Reading disability in twins. Dev. Med. Child Neurol. 15:184–187.

Bakwin, R. M., and Bakwin, H. 1948. Specific reading disability. J. Pediatr. 32:465–472.

Baldessarini, R. J. 1972. Pharmacology of the amphetamines. Pediatrics 49:694–701.

Balow, B. 1965. The long term effect of remedial reading instruction. Read. Teacher 18:581–586.

Balow, B. 1971. Perceptual-motor activities in the treatment of severe reading disability. Read. Teacher 24:513–525.

Balow, B., and Blomquist, M. 1965. Young adults ten to fifteen years after severe reading disability. Elem. School J. 66:44–48.

Balow, B., Rubin, R., and Rosen, M. J. 1975. Perinatal events as precursors of reading disability. Read. Res. Quart. 11:36–71.

Bannatyne, A. 1968. Diagnosing learning disabilities and writing remedial prescriptions. J. Learn. Disabil. 1:242–249.

Bannatyne, A. 1974. Diagnosis: A note on recategorization of the WISC scaled scores. J. Learn. Disabil. 7:272–273.

Barkley, R. A. 1977. A review of stimulant drug research with hyperactive children. J. Child Psychol. Psychiatry 18:137–165.

Barnes, E. 1951. Preface. In M. L. Shedlock, The Art of the Storyteller. Dover Publications, New York. (Originally printed in 1915.)

Bateman, B. 1969. Reading a nonmeaningful process. In L. Tarnopol (ed.), Learning Disabilities, pp. 289–304. Charles C Thomas Publisher, Springfield, Ill.

Bateson, G. 1972. Steps to an Ecology of Mind. Ballantine Books, New York.

Bateson, G. 1979. Mind and Nature. E. P. Dutton & Co., New York.

Bax, M. C. O. 1976. The assessment of the child at school entry. Pediatrics 58:403–407.

Bax, M. C. O., and Whitmore, K. 1973. Neurodevelopmental screening in the school-entrant medical examination. Lancet 2: 368–370.

Beach, F. A. 1941. Effects of brain lesions upon running activity in the male rat. J. Comp. Psychol. 31:145–149.

Beck, L., Langford, W. S., MacKay, M., and Sum, G. 1975. Childhood chemotherapy and later drug abuse and growth curve: A follow-up study of 30 adolescents. Am. J. Psychiatry 132:436–438.

Becker, W. C. 1971. Parents Are Teachers: A Child Management Program. Research Press, Champaign, Ill.

Beery, J. W. 1967. Matching of auditory and visual stimuli by average and retarded readers. Child. Dev. 38:827–833.

Bell, A. E., and Aftanas, M. S. 1972. Some correlates of reading retardation. Percept. Mot. Skills 35:659–667.

Belmont, I., and Belmont, L. 1978. Stability or change in reading achievement over time: Developmental educational implications. J. Learn. Disabil. 11:80–88.

Belmont, I., and Birch, H. G. 1974. The effect of supplemental intervention on children with low reading-readiness scores. J. Spec. Educ. 8:81–89.

Belmont, L., and Birch, H. G. 1965. Lateral dominance, lateral awareness, and reading disability. Child Dev. 36:57–71.

Bender, L. 1938. A Visual Motor Gestalt Test and Its Clinical Use. Research Monograph No. 3. American Orthopsychiatric Association, New York.

Bennett, N. 1976. Teaching Styles and Pupil Progress. Harvard University Press, Cambridge, Mass.

Benson, D. F., and Geschwind, N. 1968. Cerebral dominance and its disturbances. Pediatr. Clin. North Am. 15:759–769.

Benton, A. L. 1962. Dyslexia in relation to form perception and directional sense. In J. Money (ed.), Reading Disability: Progress and Research Needs in Dyslexia, pp. 81–102. Johns Hopkins Press, Baltimore.

Benton, A. L. 1968. Right-left discrimination. Pediatr. Clin. North Am. 15:747–758.

Benton, A. L., and Bird, J. W. 1963. The EEG and reading disability. Am. J. Orthopsychiatry 33:529–531.

Benton, A. L., and Sahs, A. L. 1968. Aspects of developmental dyslexia. Iowa Med. Soc. J. 58:377–383.

Benton, C. D. 1973. Comment: The eye and learning disabilities. J. Learn. Disabil. 6:334–336.

Bergès, J., and Lézine, I. 1965. The imitation of gestures. Clinics in Developmental Medicine No. 18. Spastics Society Medical Education and Information Unit in association with William Heinemann Medical Books, Ltd, London.

Bernstein, J. E., Page, J. G., and Janicki, R. S. 1974. Some characteristics of children with minimal brain dysfunction. In C. K. Conners (ed.), Clinical Use of Stimulant Drugs in Children, pp. 24–35. Excerpta Medica, Amsterdam.

Bettman, J. W., Jr., Stern, E. L., Whitsell, L. J., and Gofmann, H. F. 1967. Cerebral dominance in developmental dyslexia: Role of ophthalmologist. Arch. Ophthalmol. 78:722–729.

Bierman, C. W., and Furukawa, C. T. 1978. Food additives and hyperkinesis: Are there nuts among the berries? Pediatrics 61: 932–934.

Birch, H. G., and Belmont, L. 1964. Auditory-visual integration in normal and retarded readers. Am. J. Orthopsychiatry 34:852–861.

Birch, H. G., and Lefford, A. 1963. Intrasensory development in children. Monogr. Soc. Res. Child Dev. 28(5):1–48.

Bjerre, I., and Hansen, E. 1976. Psychomotor development and school adjustment of seven-year-old children with low birthweight. Acta Paediatr. Scand. 65:88–96.

Black, F. W. 1974. WISC verbal-performance discrepancies as indicators of neurologic dysfunction in pediatric patients. J. Clin. Psychol. 30:165–167.

Black, P., Jeffries, J. J., Blumer, D., Wellner, A., and Walker, A. E. 1969. The posttraumatic syndrome in children. In A. E. Walker, W. F. Caveness, and M. Critchley (eds.), Late Effects of Head Injury, pp. 142–149. Charles C Thomas Publisher, Springfield, Ill.

Blanchard, P. 1946. Psychoanalytic contributions to the problems of reading disabilities. Psychoanal. Stud. Child. 2:163–185.

Blank, M. 1968. Cognitive processes in auditory discrimination in normal and retarded readers. Child Dev. 39:1091–1101.

Blank, M., and Bridger, W. H. 1966. Deficiencies in verbal labeling in retarded readers. Am. J. Orthopsychiatry 36:840–847.

Blank, M., Weider, S., and Bridger, W. H. 1968. Verbal deficiencies in abstract thinking in early reading retardation. Am. J. Orthopsychiatry 38:823–834.

Blom, G. E. 1972. Sex differences in reading disability. In E. O. Calkins (ed.), Reading Forum, pp. 31–46. DHEW Publication No. (NIH) 72-44.

Bloom, B. S. 1964. Stability and Change in Human Characteristics. John Wiley & Sons, New York.

Bluestone, C. D., and Shurin, P. A. 1974. Middle ear disease in childhood: Pathogenesis, diagnosis, and management. Pediatr. Clin. North Am. 21:379–400.

Boder, E. 1971. Developmental dyslexia: Prevailing concepts and a new diagnostic approach. In H. R. Myklebust (ed.), Progress in Learning Disabilities, Vol. 2, pp. 293–321. Grune & Stratton, New York.

Boder, E. 1973. Developmental dyslexia: A diagnostic approach based on three atypical reading-spelling patterns. Dev. Med. Child Neurol. 15:663–687.

Boder, E. 1976. School failure—Evaluation and treatment. Pediatrics 58:394–403.

Bond, G. L., and Tinker, M. A. 1973. Reading Difficulties: Their Diagnosis and Correction. Prentice-Hall, Englewood Cliffs, N.J.

Borland, B. L., and Heckman, H. K. 1976. Hyperactive boys and their brothers. Arch. Gen. Psychiatry 33:669–675.

Boshes, B., and Myklebust, H. R. 1964. A neurological and behavioral study of children with learning disorders. Neurology 14: 7–12.

Botel, M., and Granowsky, A. 1972. A formula for measuring syntactic complexity: A directional effort. Elem. English 49:513–516.

Brainerd, C. J. 1973. The origins of number concepts. Sci. Am. 228(3):101–109.

Brenner, A. 1977. A study of the efficacy of the Feingold diet on hyperactive children. Clin. Pediatr. 7:652–656.

Brenner, A. 1979. Trace mineral levels in hyperactive children responding to the Feingold diet. J. Pediatr. 94:944–945.

Broudy, H. S. 1976. Ideological, political, and moral considerations in the use of drugs in hyperkinetic therapy. School Rev. 85: 43–60.

Brown, R. T., and Sleator, E. K. 1979. Methylphenidate in hyperkinetic children: Differences in dose effects on impulsive behavior. Pediatrics 64:408–411.

Bryan, T. H., and Bryan, J. H. 1975. Understanding Learning Disabilities. Alfred Publishing Co., Port Washington, N.Y.

Bryant, P. 1974. Perception and Understanding in Young Children. Basic Books, New York.

Buchsbaum, M., and Wender, P. 1973. Average evoked responses in normal and minimally brain dysfunctioned children treated with amphetamine: A preliminary report. Arch. Gen. Psychiatry 29:764–770.

Burns, R. C., and Kaufman, S. H. 1970. Kinetic Family Drawings (K-F-D): An Introduction to Understanding Children through Kinetic Drawings. Brunner/Mazel, New York.

Burns, R. C., and Kaufman, S. H. 1972. Actions, Styles and Symbols in Kinetic Family Drawings (K-F-D): An Interpretative Manual. Brunner/Mazel, New York.

Buros, O. K. (ed.). 1972. The Seventh Mental Measurements Yearbook, 2 Vols. Gryphon Press, Highland Park, N.J.

Buros, O. K. (ed.). 1974. Tests in Print, Vol. 2. Gryphon Press, Highland Park, N.J.

Byers, R. K., and McLean, W. T. 1962. Etiology and course of certain hemiplegias with aphasia in childhood. Pediatrics 29:376–383.

Calkins, E. O. (ed.). 1972. Reading Forum. NINDS Monograph No. 11, DHEW Publication No. (NIH) 72–74.

Calnan, M., and Richardson, K. 1977. Speech problems among children in a national survey—Associations with reading, general ability, mathematics and syntactic maturity. Educ. Stud. 3:55–56.

Camp, B. 1973. Learning rate and retention in retarded readers. J. Learn. Disabil. 6:65–71.

Campbell, S. B., Endman, M. W., and Bernfeld, G. 1977. A three-year follow-up of hyperactive preschoolers into elementary school. J. Child Psychol. Psychiatry 18:239–249.

Campbell, S. B., Schleifer, M., Weiss, G., and Perlman, T. 1977. A two-year follow up of hyperactive preschoolers. Am. J. Orthopsychiatry 47:149–162.

Cantwell, D. P. 1972. Psychiatric illness in the families of hyperactive children. Arch. Gen. Psychiatry 27:414–417.

Cantwell, D. P. 1977. Psychopharmacologic treatment of the minimal brain dysfunction syndrome. In J. M. Wiener (ed.), Psychopharmacology in Childhood and Adolescence, pp. 119–148. Basic Books, New York.

Cantwell, D. P. 1978. Hyperactivity and antisocial behavior. J. Am. Acad. Child Psychiatry 17:252–262.

Caplan, P. J., and Kinsbourne, M. 1976. Baby drops the rattle: Asymmetry of duration of grasp by infants. Child Dev. 47:532–534.

Capute, A. J., and Accardo, P. J. 1978. Linguistic and auditory milestones in the first two years of life: A language inventory for the practicing pediatrician. Clin. Pediatr. 17:847–853.

Capute, A. J., and Accardo, P. J. 1980. The minimal cerebral dysfunction-learning disability syndrome complex. In S. Gabel and M. Erickson (eds.), Child Development and Developmental Disabilities, pp. 287–301. Little, Brown, & Co., Boston.

Capute, A. J., Accardo, P. J., Bender, M., and Ross, A. 1980. Dyslexia: Initial assessment and outcome. J. Dev. Behav. Pediatr. 1:24–28.

Capute, A. J., Accardo, P. J., Vining, E. P. G., Rubenstein, J. E., and Harryman, S. 1978. Primitive Reflex Profile. Monographs in Developmental Pediatrics, Vol. 1. University Park Press, Baltimore.

Capute, A. J., Niedermeyer, E. F. L., and Richardson, F. 1968. The electroencephalogram in children with minimal cerebral dysfunction. Pediatrics 41:1104–1114.

Carroll, J. B. 1972. Illinois test of psycholinguistic abilities. In O. K. Buros (ed.), Seventh Mental Measurements Yearbook, Vol. 1, pp. 819–823. Gryphon Press, Highland Park, N.J.

Cashdan, A. 1969. The role of movement in language learning. In P. Wolff and R. MacKeith (eds.), Planning for Better Learning, pp. 37–42. Spastics Society Medical Education and Information Unit in association with William Heinemann Medical Books, Ltd., London.

Cashdan, A., and Pumfrey, P. D. 1969. Some effects of the remedial teaching of reaching. Educ. Res. 11:138–142.

Cashdan, A., Pumfrey, P. D., and Lunzer, E. A. 1971. Children receiving remedial teaching in reading. Educ. Res. 13:98–105.

Cassin, B. 1969. The eye and dyslexia. Am. Orthopt. J. 19:136–142.

Chalfant, J. C., and Scheffelin, M. A. 1969. Central Processing Dysfunctions in Children. DHEW Publication No. (NIH) 73-52. NINDS Monograph No. 9.

Chall, J. 1967. Learning to Read: The Great Debate. McGraw-Hill Book Co., New York.

Charlton, M. H. 1972. Minimal brain dysfunction and the hyperkinetic child: Clinical aspects. N.Y. State J. Med. 72:2058–2068.

Chase, H. P. 1973. The effects of intrauterine and postnatal undernutrition on normal brain development. Ann. N.Y. Acad. Sci. 205:231–244.

Chess, S. 1972. Neurological dysfunction and childhood behavioral pathology. J. Autism and Child. Schizophr. 2:299–311.

Chi, J. G., Dooling, E. C., and Gilles, F. H. 1977. Gyral development of the human brain. Ann. Neurol. 1:86–93.

Chomsky, C. 1970. Reading, writing, and phonology. Harvard Educ. Rev. 40:287–309.

Chomsky, N. 1973. Recent contributions to the theory of innate ideas. In S. G. Sapir and A. C. Nitzburg (eds.), Children with Learning Problems, pp. 99–108. Brunner/Mazel, New York.

Christensen, A. L. 1975. Luria's Neuropsychological Investigation. Spectrum, New York.

Clark, M. M. 1970. Reading Difficulties in Schools. Penguin Books, Baltimore.

Clements, S. D. 1966. Minimal Brain Dysfunction in Children. DHEW Publication No. (NIH) 73-349. NINDB Monograph No. 3.

Clements, S. D., and Peters, J. E. 1962. Minimal brain dysfunctions in the school-age child. Arch. Gen. Psychiatry 6:185–197.

Clements, S. D., and Peters, J. E. 1973. Psychoeducational programming for children with minimal brain dysfunctions. Ann. N.Y. Acad. Sci. 205:46–51.

Clifford, G. J. 1975. The Shape of American Education. Prentice-Hall, Englewood Cliffs, N.J.

Close, J. 1973. Scored neurological examination. Psychopharmacol. Bull. Special Issue: Pharmacotherapy of Children, pp. 142–150.

Cohen, D. J., and Young, J. G. 1977. Neurochemistry and child psychiatry. J. Am. Acad. Child Psychiatry 16:353–411.

Cohen, H. J., and Diner, H. 1970. The significance of developmental dental enamel defects in neurological diagnosis. Pediatrics 46:737–747.

Cohen, H. J., Diner, H., and Davis, J. G. 1975. Stigmata, dental defects and dermatoglyphics as aids in neurological diagnosis. Dev. Med. Child Neurol. 17:365–368.

Cohen, H. J., Taft, L. T., Mahadeviah, M. S., and Birch, H. G. 1967. Developmental changes in overflow in normal and aberrantly functioning children. J. Pediatr. 71:39–47.

Cohen, J. D. 1976. Is there a greater incidence of color-vision deficiencies in learning-disabled children? Clin. Pediatr. 15:518–522.

Cohen, R. 1961. Delayed acquisition of reading and writing abilities in children. Arch. Neurol. 4:153–164.

Cohen, S. A. 1969. Studies in visual perception and reading in disadvantaged children. J. Learn. Disabil. 2:498–507.

Cohen, S. A. 1976. The fuzziness and the flab: Some solutions to research problems in learning disabilities. J. Spec. Educ. 10:129–136.

Cohn, R. 1961. Dyscalculia. Arch. Neurol. 4:301–307.

Cohn, R. 1968. Developmental dyscalculia. Pediatr. Clin. North Am. 15:651–668.

Cohn, R. 1971. Arithmetic and learning disabilities. In H. R. Myklebust (ed.), Progress in Learning Disabilities, Vol. 2, pp. 322–389. Grune & Stratton, New York.

Colarusso, R. P., Martin, H., and Hartung, J. 1975. Specific visual perceptual skills as long-term predictors of academic success. J. Learn. Disabil. 8:651–655.

Colleran, J. M. (ed., transl.). 1950. St. Augustine. The Greatness of the Soul: The Teacher. ACW Vol. 9. Newman Press, New York.

Committee on Nutrition, American Academy of Pediatrics. 1976. Megavitamin therapy for childhood psychosis and learning disabilities. Pediatrics 58:910–912; Postgrad. Med. 61(4):230–233.

Conners, C. K. 1967. The syndrome of minimal brain dysfunction: Psychological aspects. Pediatr. Clin. North Am. 14:749–766.

Conners, C. K. 1969. A teacher rating scale to use in drug studies with children. Am. J. Psychiatry 126:884–888.

Conners, C. K. 1970. Cortical visual evoked response in children with learning disorders. Psychophysiology 7:418–428.

Conners, C. K. 1971. Recent drug studies with hyperkinetic children. J. Learn. Disabil. 4:476–483.

Conners, C. K. 1972. Psychological effects of stimulant drugs in children with minimal brain dysfunction. Pediatrics 49:702–708.

Conners, C. K. 1973. Psychological assessment of children with minimal brain dysfunction. Ann. N.Y. Acad. Sci. 205:274–302.

Conners, C. K. 1974a. The effect of pemoline and dextroamphetamine on evoked potentials under two conditions of attention. In C. K. Conners (ed.), Clinical Use of Stimulant Drugs in Children, pp. 165–178. Excerpta Medica, Amsterdam.

Conners, C. K. (ed.). 1974b. Clinical Use of Stimulant Drugs in Children. Excerpta Medica, Amsterdam.

Conners, C. K. 1977. Methodological considerations in drug research with children. In J. M. Wiener (ed.), Psychopharmacology in Childhood and Adolescence, pp. 58–83. Basic Books, New York.

Conners, C. K., Goyette, C. H., Southwick, D. A., Lees, J. M., and Andrulonis, P. A. 1976. Food additives and hyperkinesis: A controlled double-blind experiment. Pediatrics 58:154–166.

Conners, C. K., Rothschild, G. H., Eisenberg, L., Stone, L., and Robinson, E. 1969. Dextroamphetamine in children with learning disorders. Arch. Gen. Psychiatry 21:182–190.

Connolly, K., and Stratton, P. 1968. Developmental changes in associated movements. Dev. Med. Child Neurol. 10:49–56.

Conrad, W. G., and Insel, J. 1967. Anticipating the response to amphetamine therapy in the treatment of hyperkinetic children. Pediatrics 40:96–99.

Cooper, F. S. 1972. How is language conveyed by speech? In J. F. Kavanagh and I. G. Mattingly (eds.), Language by Ear and by Eye, pp. 25–45. MIT Press, Cambridge, Mass.

Cooper, J. R., Bloom, F. E., and Roth, R. H. 1974. The Biochemical Basis of Neuropharmacology. Oxford University Press, New York.

Corrigan, F. V., Berger, S. I., Dienstbier, R. A., and Strok, E. S. 1967. The influence of prematurity on school performance. Am. J. Ment. Defic. 71:533–535.

Corson, S. A., Corson, E. O'L., Kirilcuk, V., and Arnold, L. E. 1971. Tranquilizing effects of d-amphetamine on hyperkinetic untrainable dogs. Fed. Proc. 30:206.

Cott, A. 1971. Orthomolecular approach to the treatment of learning disabilities. Schizophrenia 3:95–105.

Council on Child Health. 1975. Medication for hyperkinetic children. Pediatrics 55:560–562.

Cowgill, M., Friedland, S., and Shapiro, R. 1973. Predicting learning disabilities from kindergarten reports. J. Learn. Disabil. 6: 577–582.

Critchley, M. 1963. The problem of developmental dyslexia. Proc. Roy. Soc. Med. 56:209–212.

Critchley, M. 1968. Dysgraphia and other anomalies of written speech. Pediatr. Clin. North Am. 15:639–650.

Critchley, M. 1970. The Dyslexic Child. Charles C Thomas Publisher, Springfield, Ill.

Cronbach, L. J. 1970. Essentials of Psychological Testing. Harper & Row, New York.

Crook, W. G. 1974a. The allergic tension-fatigue syndrome. Pediatr. Ann. 3(10):69–77.

Crook, W. G. 1974b. An alternative method of managing the hyperactive child. Pediatrics 54:656.

Crook, W. G. 1975. Food allergy—The great masquerader. Pediatr. Clin. North Am. 22:227–238.

Croxton, F. E. 1959. Elementary Statistics with Applications in Medicine and the Biological Sciences. Dover Publications, New York.

Cruickshank, W. M. 1977. Least-restrictive placement: Administrative wishful thinking. J. Learn. Disabil. 10:193–194.

Curr, W., and Gourlay, N. 1953. An experimental evaluation of remedial education. Br. J. Educ. Psychol. 23:45–55.

Dalby, J. T., Kinsbourne, M., Swanson, J. M., and Sobol, M. P. 1977. Hyperactive children's underuse of learning time: Correction by stimulant treatment. Child Dev. 48:1448–1453.

Daryn, E. 1961. Problems of children with diffuse brain damage. Arch. Gen. Psychiatry 4:299–306.

David, G. D. 1958. Caudate lesions and spontaneous locomotion in the monkey. Neurology 8:135–139.

David, O., Clark, J., and Voeller, K. 1972. Lead and hyperactivity. Lancet 2:900–903.

David, O. J., Hoffman, S. P., Sverd, J., Clark, J., and Voeller, K. 1976. Lead and hyperactivity. Behavioral response to chelation. A pilot study. Am. J. Psychiatry 133:1155–1158.

de Beer, G. 1958. Embryos and Ancestors. Oxford University Press, New York.

De Cecco, J. P. 1968. The Psychology of Learning and Instruction: Educational Psychology. Prentice-Hall, Englewood Cliffs, N.J.

de Hirsch, K. 1973. Early language development and minimal brain dysfunction. Ann. N.Y. Acad. Sci. 205:158–164.

de Hirsch, K., Jansky, J. J., and Langford, W. S. 1966. Predicting Reading Failure: A Preliminary Study. Harper & Row, New York.

Deibert, A. N., and Harmon, A. J. 1973. New Tools for Changing Behavior. Research Press, Champaign, Ill.

de la Burdé, B., and Choate, M. S. 1975. Early asymptomatic lead exposure and development at school age. J. Pediatr. 87:638–642.

Delacato, C. H. 1959. The Treatment and Prevention of Reading Problems. Charles C Thomas Publishers, Springfield, Ill.

Delacato, C. H. 1963. The Diagnosis and Treatment of Speech and Reading Problems. Charles C Thomas Publisher, Springfield, Ill.

Delacato, C. H. 1966. Neurological Organization and Reading. Charles C Thomas Publisher, Springfield, Ill.

Demerdash, A., Eeg-Olofsson, O., and Petersen, I. 1968. The incidence of 14 and 6 per second positive spikes in the population of normal children. Dev. Med. Child Neurol. 10:309–316.

Denburg, M. L. (ed.). 1972. Readings for the Psychology of the Exceptional Child: Emphasis on Learning Disabilities. MSS Information Corporation, New York.

Denckla, M. B. 1972. Clinical syndromes in learning disabilities: The case for "splitting" vs. "lumping." J. Learn. Disabil. 5: 401–406.

Denckla, M. B. 1973. Development of speed in repetitive and successive finger-movements in normal children. Dev. Med. Child Neurol. 15:635–645.

Denckla, M. B., and Rudel, R. G. 1978. Anomalies of motor development in hyperactive boys. Ann. Neurol. 3:231–233.

Denenberg, V. H., Garbanati, J., Sherman, G., Yutzey, D. A., and Kaplan, R. 1978. Infantile stimulation induces brain lateralization in rats. Science 201:1150–1151.

Denhoff, E. 1973a. The hyperkinetic behavior syndrome: Clinical reflections. Pediatr. Ann. 2(5):15–28.

Denhoff, E. 1973b. The natural life history of children with minimal brain dysfunction. Ann. N.Y. Acad. Sci. 205:188–205.

Denhoff, E. 1976. Learning disabilities: An office approach. Pediatrics 58:409–411.

Denhoff, E., Davids, A., and Hawkins, R. 1971. Effects of dextroamphetamine on hyperkinetic children: A controlled double blind study. J. Learn. Disabil. 4:491–498.

Denhoff, E., Hainsworth, P. K., and Hainsworth, M. L. 1972. The child at risk for learning disorder. Clin. Pediatr. 11:164–170.

Denhoff, E., Hainsworth, P. K., and Siqueland, M. L. 1968. The measurement of psychoneurological factors contributing to learning efficiency. J. Learn. Disabil. 1:636–644.

Denhoff, E., Siqueland, M. L., Komich, M. P., and Hainsworth, P. K. 1968. Developmental and predictive characteristics of items from the Meeting Street School Screening Test. Dev. Med. Child Neurol. 10:220–232.

Denson, R., Nanson, J. L., and McWatters, M. A. 1975. Hyper-kinesis and maternal smoking. Can. Psychiatric Assoc. J. 20: 183–187.

Deonna, T., Beaumanoir, A., Gaillard, F., and Assal, G. 1977. Ac-quired aphasia in childhood with seizure disorder: A heterogene-ous syndrome. Neuropädiatrie 8:263–273.

de Quiros, J. B. 1976. Diagnosis of vestibular disorders in the learning disabled. J. Learn. Disabil. 9:39–47.

Derby, B. M. 1972. Minimal brain dysfunction and the hyper-kinetic child: Structural basis. N.Y. State J. Med. 72:2061–2062.

Desmond, M. M., Vorderman, A. L., and Fisher E. S. 1978. As-sessment of learning competence during the pediatric examina-tion. Curr. Probl. Pediatr. 8(8).

Dickens, C. 1944. Nicholas Nickleby. Dodd, Mead & Co., New York. (Originally printed in 1839.)

DiLeo, J. H. 1970. Young Children and Their Drawings. Brunner/Mazel, New York.

DiLeo, J. H. 1973. Children's Drawings as Diagnostic Aids. Brun-ner/Mazel, New York.

Dineen, J. P., Clark, H. B., and Risley, T. R. 1977. Peer tutoring among elementary students: Educational benefits to the tutor. J. Appl. Behav. Anal. 10:231–238.

Doehring, D. G. 1976. Acquisition of rapid reading responses. Monogr. Soc. Res. Child Dev. 41(2) (serial no. 165).

Doman, G. 1964. How to Teach Your Baby to Read: The Gentle Revolution. Random House, New York.

The Doman-Delacato treatment of neurologically handicapped children. 1968. Arch. Phys. Med. Rehab. 49:183–186.

Downing, J. (ed.). 1973. Comparative Reading: Cross-National Studies of Behavior and Processes in Reading and Writing. Macmillan Publishing Co., New York.

Drew, A. L. 1956. A neurological appraisal of familial congenital word-blindness. Brain 79:440–460.

Dubey, D. R. 1976. Organic factors in hyperkinesis: A critical evaluation. Am. J. Orthopsychiatry 46:353–366.

Dubey, D. R., and Kaufman, K. F. 1978. Home management of hyperkinetic children. J. Pediatr. 93:141–146.

Dubowitz, L. M. S., Leibowitz, D., and Goldberg, C. 1977. A clini-cal screening test for assessment of intellectual development in four- and five-year-old children. Dev. Med. Child Neurol. 19: 776–782.

Duffy, F. H., Burchfiel, J. L., and Lombroso, C. T. 1979. Brain electrical activity mapping (BEAM): A method for extending the clinical utility of EEG and evoked potential data. Ann. Neurol. 5:309–321.

Durrell, D. D. 1955. Durrell Analysis of Reading Difficulty. Harcourt, Brace & World, New York.

Dykman, R. A., Ackerman, P. T., Clements, S. D., and Peters, J. E. 1971. Specific learning disabilities: An attentional deficit syndrome. In H. R. Myklebust (ed.), Progress in Learning Disabilities, Vol. 2, pp. 56–93. Grune & Stratton, New York.

Dykman, R. A., Ackerman, P. T., Peters, J. E., and McGrew, J. 1974. Psychological tests. In C. K. Conners (ed.), Clinical Use of Stimulant Drugs in Children, pp. 44–52. Excerpta Medica, Amsterdam.

Dykman, R. A., Peters, J. E., and Ackerman, P. T. 1973. Experimental approaches to the study of minimal brain dysfunction: A follow-up study. Ann. N.Y. Acad. Sci. 205:93–108.

Eames, T. H. 1948. Comparison of eye conditions among 1,000 reading failures, 500 ophthalmic patients and 150 unselected children. Am. J. Ophthalmol. 31:713–717.

Eames, T. H. 1962. Physical factors in reading. Read. Teacher 15: 427–432.

Edwards, D. 1969. Meihem in ce klasrum. In R. A. Baker (ed.), A Stress Analysis of a Strapless Evening Gown and Other Essays for a Scientific Age, pp. 125–129. Anchor Books, New York.

Egan, D. F., Illingworth, R. S., and MacKeith, R. C. 1969. Developmental Screening 0–5 Years. Clinics in Developmental Medicine No. 30. Spastics Society Medical Education and Information Unit in association with William Heinemann Medical Books, Ltd., London.

Eisenberg, L. 1959. Office evaluation of specific reading disability in children. Pediatrics 23:997–1003.

Eisenberg, L. 1966a. The epidemiology of reading retardation and a program for preventive intervention. In J. Money (ed.), The Disabled Reader: Education of the Dyslexic Child, pp. 3–19. Johns Hopkins Press, Baltimore.

Eisenberg, L. 1966b. The management of the hyperkinetic child. Dev. Med. Child Neurol. 8:593–598.

Eisenberg, L. 1971. Principles of drug therapy in child psychiatry with special reference to stimulant drugs. Am. J. Orthopsychiatry 41:371-279.

Eisenberg, L. 1972. The clinical use of stimulant drugs in children. Pediatrics 49:709-715.

Eisenberg, L. 1978. Hyperkinesis revisited. Pediatrics 61:319-321.

Eisenson, J. 1969. Developmental aphasia: Therapeutic implications. In P. Wolff and R. MacKeith (eds.), Planning for Better Learning, pp. 100-107. Spastics Society Medical Education and Information Unit in association with William Heinnemann Medical Books, Ltd., London.

Eleftheriou, B. E., and Boehlke, K. W. 1967. Brain monoamine oxidase in mice after exposure to aggression and defeat. Science 155:1693-1694.

Eliasson, S. G., Prensky, A. L., and Hardin, W. B. 1974. Neurological Pathophysiology. Oxford University Press, New York.

Elkonin, D. B. 1973. U.S.S.R. In J. Downing (ed.), Comparative Reading, pp. 551-559. Macmillan Publishing Co., New York.

Englehardt, W. 1975. Die validität des Frostig Developmental Test of Visual Perception (DTVP). [The validity of the Frostig Developmental Test of Visual Perception (DTVP).] Z. Entwicklungpsychol. Pädagog. Psychol. 7:100-112.

Epstein, L. C., Lasagna, L., Conners, C. K., and Rodriguez, A. 1968. Correlation of dextroamphetamine excretion and drug response in hyperkinetic children. J. Nerv. Ment. Dis. 146:136-146.

Erenberg, G. J. 1972. Drug therapy in minimal brain dysfunction: A commentary. J. Pediatr. 81:359-365.

Erenberg, G. 1973. Treatment of the hyperactive child. Pediatr. Ann. 2(5):56-79.

Erickson, M. T. 1975. The Z-score discrepancy method for identifying reading disabled children. J. Learn. Disabil. 8:308-312.

Erickson, M. T. 1977. Reading disability in relation to performance on neurological tests for minimal brain dysfunction. Dev. Med. Child Neurol. 19:768-775.

Farnham-Diggory, S. 1978. Learning Disabilities: A Psychological Perspective. Harvard University Press, Cambridge, Mass.

Federici, L., Sims, H., and Bashian, A. 1976. Use of Meeting Street School Screening Test and the Myklebust pupil rating scale with first-grade black urban children. Psychol. Schools 13:386–389.

Fedio, P., and Mirsky, A. F. 1969. Selective intellectual deficits in children with temporal lobe or centrencephalic epilepsy. Neuropsychologia 7:287–300.

Feingold, B. 1975a. Hyperkinesis and learning disabilities linked to artificial food flavors and colors. Am. J. Nurs. 75:797–803.

Feingold, B. F. 1975b. Why Is Your Child Hyperactive? Random House, New York.

Feingold, B. F. 1976. Hyperkinesis and learning disabilities linked to ingestion of artificial food colors and flavors. J. Learn. Disabil. 9:551–559.

Feingold, M., and Bossert, W. H. 1974. Normal values for selected physical parameters: An aid to syndrome delineation. Birth Defects, Original Article Series 10:13.

Fernald, G. M . 1943. Remedial Techniques in Basic School Subjects. McGraw-Hill Book Co., New York.

Fink, M., and Bender, M. B. 1953. Perception of simultaneous tactile stimuli in normal children. Neurology 3:27–34.

Finlayson, M. A. J., and Reitan, R. M. 1976. Tactile-perceptual functioning in relation to intellectual, cognitive and reading skills in younger and older normal children. Dev. Med. Child Neurol. 18:442–446.

Finocchiaro, A. C. J. 1974. Behavior characteristics in learning-disabled children with postural reflex dysfunction. Am. J. Occup. Ther. 28:30–34.

Firestone, P., Davey, J., Goodman, J. T., and Peters, S. 1978. The effects of caffeine and methylphenidate on hyperactive children. J. Am. Acad. Child Psychiatry 17:445–456.

Firestone, P., Lewy, F., and Douglas, V. I. 1976. Hyperactivity and physical anomalies. Can. Psychiatric Assoc. J. 21:23–26.

Firestone, P., Poitras-Wright, H., and Douglas, V. 1978. The effects of caffeine on hyperactive children. J. Learn. Disabil. 11:133–141.

Fish, B. 1971. The "one child, one drug" myth of stimulants in hyperkinesis: Importance of diagnostic categories in evaluating treatment. Arch. Gen. Psychiatry 25:193–203.

Fitzhardinge, P. M., and Steven, E. M. 1972. The small-for-date infant. II. Neurological and intellectual sequelae. Pediatrics 50:50–57.

Flax, N. 1973. The eye and learning disabilities. J. Learn. Disabil. 6:328–333.

Flesch, R. 1948. A new readability yardstick. J. Appl. Psychol. 32:221–233.

Flesch, R. 1956. Why Johnny Can't Read and What You Can Do about It. Popular Library, New York.

Flower, R. M. 1965. Auditory disorders and reading disorders. In R. M. Flower, H. F. Gofman, and L. I. Lawson (eds.), Reading Disorders: A Multidisciplinary Symposium, pp. 81–102. F. A. Davis Co., Philadelphia.

Flower, R. M., Gofman, H. F., and Lawson, L. I. (eds.). 1965. Reading Disorders: A Multidisciplinary Symposium. F. A. Davis Co., Philadelphia.

Flynn, N., and Rapoport, J. 1976. Hyperactivity in open and traditional classroom environments. J. Spec. Ed. 10:285–290.

Fog, E., and Fog, M. 1963. Cerebral inhibition examined by associated movements. In R. MacKeith and M. Bax (eds.), Minimal Cerebral Dysfunction, pp. 52–57. Spastics Society Medical Education and Information Unit in association with William Heinemann Medical Books, Ltd., London.

Forman, P. M. 1975. Pharmacological intervention. In H. R. Myklebust (ed.), Progress in Learning Disabilities, Vol. 3, pp. 151–160. Grune & Stratton, New York.

Forster, F. M. 1975. Reading epilepsy, musicogenic epilepsy, and related disorders. In H. R. Myklebust (ed.), Progress in Learning Disabilities, Vol. 3, pp. 161–177. Grune & Stratton, New York.

Foster, G. G., Schmidt, C. R., and Sabatino, D. 1976. Teacher expectancies and the label "learning disabilities." J. Learn. Disabil. 9:111–114.

Fraiberg, S. H. 1977. Insights from the Blind. Basic Books, New York.

Francis-Williams, J. 1976. Early identification of children likely to have specific learning difficulties: Report of a follow-up. Dev. Med. Child Neurol. 18:71–77.

Frank, J., and Levinson, H. 1973. Dysmetric dyslexia and dyspraxia. J. Am. Acad. Child Psychiatry 12:690–701.

Fransella, F., and Gerver, D. 1966. Multiple regression equations for predicting reading age from chronological age and WISC verbal IQ. Br. J. Educ. Psychol. 35:86–89.

Franuenheim, J. G. 1978. Academic achievement characteristics of adult males who were diagnosed as dyslexic in childhood. J. Learn. Disabil. 11:476–483.

Freeman, R. D. 1976. Minimal brain dysfunction, hyperactivity, and learning disorders: Epidemic or episode? School Rev. 85:5–30.

Friedman, R., Dale, E. P., and Wagner, J. H. 1973. Long-term comparison of 2 treatment regimens for minimal brain dysfunction. Clin. Pediatr. 12:666–671.

Frostig, M. 1965a. Corrective reading in the classroom. Read. Teacher 18:573–580.

Frostig, M. 1965b. Teaching reading to children with perceptual disturbances. In R. M. Flower, H . F. Gofman, and L. I. Lawson (eds.), Reading Disorders: A Multidisciplinary Symposium, pp. 113–127. F. A. Davis Co., Philadelphia.

Frostig, M. 1972. Visual perception, integrative functions and academic learning. J. Learn. Disabil. 5:5–15.

Frostig, M., and Maslow, P . 1969. Visual perception and early education. In L. Tarnopol (ed.), Learning Disabilities, pp. 217–237. Charles C Thomas Publisher, Springfield, Ill.

Frostig, M., and Orpet, R. E. 1969. Four approaches to the diagnosis of perceptual disturbances in reading disability. Br. J. Disord. Commun. 4:41–45.

Fry, E. 1968. Readability formula that saves time. J. Read. 11: 513–516, 575–578.

Fry, M. A., Johnson, C. S., and Muehl, S. 1970. Oral language production in relation to reading achievement among select second graders. In D. J. Bakker and P. Satz (eds.), Specific Reading Disability, pp. 123–146. Rotterdam University Press, Rotterdam.

Fuller, P. W. 1978. Attention and the EEG alpha rhythm in learning disabled children. J. Learn. Disabil. 11:303–312.

Furth, H. G. 1971. Linguistic deficiency and thinking: Research with deaf subjects 1964–1969. Psychol. Bull. 76:58–72.

Galaburda, A. M., Le May, M., Kemper, T. L., and Geschwind, N. 1978. Right-left asymmetries in the brain. Science 199:852–856.

Galambos, R. G., and Hecox, K. 1978. Clinical applications of the auditory brainstem response. Otolaryngol. Clin. North Am. 11: 709–722.

Gardner, R. 1966. The Child's Book about Brain Injury. Association for Brain Injured Children, New York.

Gardner, R. A. 1973. MBD: The Family Book about Minimal Brain Dysfunction. Jason Aronson, New York.

Garfield, J. C. 1964. Motor impersistence in normal and brain-damaged children. Neurology 14:623–630.

Garrard, S. 1973. Role of the pediatrician in the management of learning disorders. Pediatr. Clin. North Am. 20:737–754.

Garrettson, L. K., Perel, J. M., and Dayton, P. G. 1969. Methylphenidate interaction with both anticonvulsants and ethyl biscoumacetate. JAMA 207:2053–2056.

Gascon, G., Victor, D., Lombroso, C. T., and Goodglass, H. 1973. Language disorder, convulsive disorder, and electroencephalographic abnormalities. Arch. Neurol. 28:156–162.

Gerstmann, J. 1940. Syndrome of finger agnosia, disorientation for right and left, agraphia and acalculia; local diagnostic value. Arch. Neurol. Psychiatry 44:398–408.

Geschwind, N. 1962. The anatomy of acquired disorders of reading. In J. Money (ed.), Reading Disability: Progress and Research Needs in Dyslexia, pp. 115–129. Johns Hopkins Press, Baltimore.

Geschwind, N. 1965. Disconnexion syndrome in animals and man. Brain 88:237–294, 585–644.

Geschwind, N. 1968. Neurological foundations of language. In H. R. Myklebust (ed.), Progress in Learning Disabilities, Vol. 1, pp. 182–198. Grune & Stratton, New York.

Geschwind, N. 1972. Language and the brain. Sci. Am. 226(4):76–83.

Geschwind, N., and Fusillo, M. 1966. Color-naming defects in association with alexia. Arch. Neurol. 15:137–146.

Geschwind, N., and Levitsky, W. 1968. Human brain: Left-right asymmetries in temporal speech region. Science 161:186–187.

Gibson, E. J., and Levin, H. 1975. The Psychology of Reading. MIT Press, Cambridge, Mass.

Gibson, E. J., Shurcliff, A., and Yonas, A. 1970. Utilization of spelling patterns by deaf and hearing subjects. In H. Levin and J. Williams (eds.), Basic Studies on Reading, pp. 57–73. Basic Books, New York.

Ginsburg, G. P., and Hartwick, A. 1971. Directional confusion as a sign of dyslexia. Percept. Mot. Skills 32:535–543.

Ginzberg, E. 1979. The professionalization of the U.S. labor force.

Sci. Am. 240(3):48–53.

Gittelman-Klein, R. 1974. Pilot clinical trial of imipramine in hyperkinetic children. In C. K. Conners (ed.), Clinical Use of Stimulant Drugs in Children, pp. 192–201. Excerpta Medica, Amsterdam.

Gittelman-Klein, R., and Klein, D. 1976. Methylphenidate effects in learning disabilities. Arch. Gen. Psychiatry 33:655–664.

Glaser, K., and Clemmens, R. L. 1965. School failure. Pediatrics 35:128–141.

Glick, S. D., and Milloy, S. 1963. Rate-dependent effects of d-amphetamine on locomotor activity in mice: Possible relationship to paradoxical amphetamine sedation in minimal brain dysfunction. Eur. J. Pharmacol. 24:266–268.

Gofman, H. F. 1965. The identification and evaluation of children with reading disorders: A pediatrician's view. In R. M. Flower, H. F. Gofman, and L. I. Lawson (eds.), Reading Disorders: A Multidisciplinary Symposium, pp. 5–18. F. A. Davis Co., Philadelphia.

Gofman, H. F., and Allmond, B. W., Jr., 1971a. Learning and language disorders in children. I. The preschool child. Curr. Probl. Pediatr. 1(10).

Gofman, H. F., and Allmond, B. W., Jr. 1971b. Learning and language disorders in children. II. The school-age child. Curr. Probl. Pediatr. 1(11).

Goldberg, H. K., and Arnott, W. 1970. Ocular motility in learning disabilities. J. Learn. Disabil. 3:160–162.

Goldberg, H. K., and Guthrie, J. T. 1972. Evaluation of visual perceptual factors in reading disability. J. Pediatr. Ophthalmol. 9:18–25.

Goldman, P. S., Crawford, H. T., Stokes, L. P., Galkin, T. W., and Rosvold, H . E. 1974. Sex dependent behavioral effects of cerebral cortical lesions in the developing Rhesus monkey. Science 186:540–542.

Gollay, E., and Bennett, A. 1976. The College Guide for Students with Disabilities. Abt Associates, Cambridge, Mass.

Golter, M., and Michaelson, I. A. 1975. Growth, behavior, and brain catecholamines in lead-exposed neonatal rats: A reappraisal. Science 187:359–361.

Gomez, M. R. 1967. Minimal cerebral dysfunction (Maximal neurologic confusion). Clin. Pediatr. 6:589–591.

Goodenough, F. L. 1926. Measurement of Intelligence by Drawings. Harcourt, Brace & World, New York.

Goodman, K. S. 1967. Reading: A psycholinguistic guessing game. J. Read. Spec. 6:126–135.

Goodnow, J. 1977. Children Drawing. Harvard University Press, Cambridge, Mass.

Goodwin, W. C., Jr., and Erickson, M. T. 1973. Developmental problems and dental morphology. Am. J. Ment. Defic. 78:199–204.

Gottesman, R., Belmont, I., and Kaminer, R. 1975. Admission and follow-up status of reading disabled children referred to a medical clinic. J. Learn. Disabil. 8:642–650.

Goyette, G. H., Connors, C. K., Petti, T. A., and Curtis, L. E. 1978. Effects of artificial colors on hyperkinetic children: A double-blind challenge study. Psychopharmacol. Bull. 14(2):39–40.

Grande, L. M. 1962. Twelve Virtues of a Good Teacher. Sheed & Ward, New York.

Grant, W. W., Boelsche, A. N., and Zin, D. 1973. Developmental patterns of two motor functions. Dev. Med. Child Neurol. 15:171–177.

Gray, W. S. 1955. Current reading problems: A world view. Educ. Dig. 21:28–31.

Gray, W. S. 1963. Gray Oral Reading Tests. Bobbs-Merrill Co., Indianapolis.

Greenberg, L. M., Deem, M. A., and McMahon, S. 1972. Effects of dextroamphetamine, chlorpromazine, and hydroxyzine on behavior and performance in hyperactive children. Am. J. Psychiatry 129:532–539.

Greenhill, L. L., Rieder, D. O., Wender, P. H., Buchsbaum, M., and Zahn, T. P. 1973. Lithium carbonate in the treatment of hyperactive children. Arch. Gen. Psychiatry 28:636–640.

Gregory, R. L. 1974. Concepts and Mechanisms of Perception. Charles Scribner's Sons, New York.

Gross, M. D. 1976. Growth of hyperkinetic children taking methylphenidate, dextroamphetamine, or imipramine/desipramine. Pediatrics 58:423–431.

Grünewald-Zuberbier, E., Grünewald, G., and Rasche, A. 1975. Hyperactive behavior and EEG arousal reactions in children. Electroencephalogr. Clin. Neurophysiol. 38:149–159.

Guay, R. B., and McDaniel, E. D. 1977. The relationship between mathematics achievement and spatial abilities among elementary school children. J. Res. Math. Educ. 8:211–215.

Gubbay, S. S., Ellis, E., Walton, J. N., and Court, S. D. M. 1965. Clumsy children: A study of apraxic and agnosic defects in 21 children. Brain 88:295–312.

Guey, J., Charles, C., Coquery, C., Roger, J., and Soulayrol, R. 1967. Study of the psychological effects of ethosuximide (Zarontin) on 25 children suffering from *petit mal* epilepsy. Epilepsia 8:129–141.

Guthrie, J. T. 1973. Reading comprehension and syntactic responses in good and poor readers. J. Educ. Psychol. 65:294–299.

Guthrie, J. T., and Goldberg, H. K. 1972. Visual sequential memory in reading disability. J. Learn. Disabil. 5:41–46.

Guyer, B. L., and Friedman, M. P. 1975. Hemispheric processing and cognitive styles in learning-disabled and normal children. Child Dev. 46:658–668.

Haeussermann, E. 1958. Developmental Potential of Preschool Children. Grune & Stratton, New York.

Hall, R. A., Griffin, R. B., Myer, D. L., Hopkins, K. H., and Rappaport, M. 1976. Evoked potential, stimulus intensity and drug treatment in hyperkinesis. Psychophysiology 13:405–418.

Hallgren, B. 1950. Specific dyslexia ("Congenital word-blindness"): A clinical and genetic study. Acta Psychiatr. Neurol. Scand. Suppl. 65:1–287.

Halliday, R., Rosenthal, J. H., Naylor, H., and Callaway, E. 1976. Averaged evoked potential predictors of clinical improvement in hyperactive children treated with methylphenidate: An initial study and replication. Psychophysiology 13:429–440.

Halverson, C. F., Jr., and Victor, J. B. 1976. Minor physical anomalies and problem behavior in elementary school children. Child Dev. 47:281–285.

Hammill, D. D. 1972. Training visual perceptual processes. J. Learn. Disabil. 5:552–559.

Hammill, D. D., and Larsen, S. C. 1974a. The effectiveness of psycholinguistic training. Except. Child. 41:5–14.

Hammill, D. D., and Larsen, S. C. 1974b. The relationship of selected auditory perceptual skills and reading ability. J. Learn. Disabil. 7:429–435.

Hammill, D. D., and Larsen, S. C. 1978. The effectiveness of psycholinguistic training: A reaffirmation of position. Except. Child. 44:402–414.

Hanshaw, J. B., Scheiner, A. P., Moxley, A. W., Gaev, L., Abel,

V., and Scheiner, B. 1976. School failure and deafness after "silent" congenital cytomegalovirus infection. New Engl. J. Med. 295:468-470.

Hardin, W. B., Jr., and Merson, R. M. 1974. The higher-order dysfunctions: Apraxia, agnosia, and aphasia. In S. G. Eliasson, A. L. Prensky, and W. B. Hardin, Jr. (eds.), Neurological Pathophysiology, pp. 170-186. Oxford University Press, New York.

Haring, N. G., and Ridgway, R. W. 1967. Early identification of children with learning disabilities. Except. Child. 33:387-395.

Harley, J. P., Matthews, C. G., and Eichman, P. 1978. Synthetic food colors and hyperactivity in children: A double-blind challenge experiment. Pediatrics 62:975-983.

Harley, J. P., Ray, R. S., Tomasi, L., Eichman, P. L., Matthews, C. G., Chun, R., Cleeland, C. S., and Traisman, E. 1978. Hyperkinesis and food additives: Testing the Feingold hypothesis. Pediatrics 61:818-828.

Harris, A. J. 1957. Lateral dominance, directional confusion, and reading disability. J. Psychol. 44:283-294.

Harris, A. J. 1970. How to Increase Reading Ability: A Guide to Developmental and Remedial Methods. David McKay, New York.

Harris, A. J., and Roswell, F. G. 1953. Clinical diagnosis of reading disability. J. Psychol. 36:323-340.

Harris, A. J., and Sipay, E. R. 1975. How to Increase Reading Ability: A Guide to Developmental and Remedial Methods. David McKay, New York.

Harris, D. B., 1963. Children's Drawings As Measures of Intellectual Maturity: A Revision and Extension of the Goodenough Draw-a-Man Test. Harcourt, Brace & World, New York.

Harris, D. B., Roberts, J., and Pinder, G. D. 1970. Intellectual Maturity of Children As Measured by the Goodenough-Harris Drawing Test. Public Health Service Publication No. 1000, Series 11, No. 105.

Harris, L. J. 1978. Sex differences in spatial ability: Possible environmental, genetic, and neurological factors. In M. Kinsbourne (ed.), Asymmetrical Function of the Brain, pp. 405-522. Cambridge University Press, New York.

Hart, Z., Rennick, P. M., Klinge, V., and Schwartz, M. L. 1974. A pediatric neurologist's contribution to evaluations of school underachievers. Am. J. Dis. Child. 128:319-323.

Hartlage, L. C. 1979. Learning disabilities. In P. R. Nader (ed.), School-Related Health Care, pp. 28-33. Report of the Ninth Ross Roundtable on Critical Approaches to Common Pediatric Problems. Ross Laboratories, Columbus, Oh.

Hartlage, L. C., and Green, J. B. 1973. The EEG as a predictor of intellective and academic performance. J. Learn. Disabil. 6:239-242.

Hartlage, L. C., and Lucas, D. G. 1973. Mental Development Evaluation of the Pediatric Patient. Charles C Thomas Publisher, Springfield, Ill.

Hartstein, J. (ed.). 1971. Current Concepts in Dyslexia. C. V. Mosby Co., Saint Louis.

Harvey, D. H. P., and Marsh, R. W. 1978. The effects of de-caffeinated coffee versus whole coffee on hyperactive children. Dev. Med. Child Neurol. 20:81-86.

Havighurst, R. J. 1976. Choosing a middle path for the use of drugs with hyperactive children. School Rev. 85:61-77.

Hechtman, L., Weiss, G., Finklestein, J., Werner, A., and Benn, R. 1976. Hyperactives as young adults: Preliminary report. Can. Med. Assoc. J. 115:625-630.

Hechtman, L., Weiss, G., and Metrakos, K. 1978. Hyperactive individuals as young adults: Current and longitudinal electroencephalographic evaluation and its relation to outcome. Can. Med. Assoc. J. 118:919-923.

Hechtman, L., Weiss, G., and Perlman, T. 1978. Growth and cardiovascular measures in hyperactive individuals as young adults and in matched normal controls. Can. Med. Assoc. J. 118: 1247-1250.

Heim, A. 1970. Intelligence and Personality. Penguin Books, Baltimore.

Heller, T. M. 1963. Word blindness—A survey of the literature and a report of twenty-eight cases. Pediatrics 31:669-691.

Henderson, A. G. 1975. Electrophysiological tests of hearing. Dev. Med. Child Neurol. 17:96-99.

Hermann, K. 1959. Reading Disability. Munksgaard, Copenhagen.

Hertzig, M. D., Bortner, M., and Birch, H. G. 1969. Neurological findings in children educationally designated as "brain damaged." Am. J. Orthopsychiatry 39:437-446.

Hertzig, S. A., Birch, H. G., Richardson, S. A., and Tizard, J.

1972. Intellectual levels of school children severely malnourished during the first two years of infancy. Pediatrics 49:814–824.

Hier, D. B., LeMay, M., Rosenberger, P. B., and Perlo, V. P. 1978. Developmental dyslexia: Evidence for a subgroup with a reversal of cerebral asymmetry. Arch. Neurol. 35:90–92.

Hinshelwood, J. 1917. Congenital Word-Blindness. H. K. Lewis & Co., Ltd., London.

Hiscock, M., and Kinsbourne, M. 1978. Ontogeny of cerebral dominance: Evidence from time-sharing asymmetry in children. Dev. Psychol. 14:321–329.

Hodges, W. F., and Spielberg, C. D. 1969. Digit span: An indication of trait or state anxiety? J. Consult. Clin. Psychol. 33:430–434.

Holm, V. A., and Kunze, L. H. 1969. Effect of chronic otitis media on language and speech development. Pediatrics 43:833–839.

Huelsman, C. B., Jr. 1970. The WISC subtest syndrome for disabled readers. Percept. Mot. Skills 30:535–550.

Huessy, H. R., and Cohen, A. H. 1976. Hyperkinetic behaviors and learning disabilities followed over seven years. Pediatrics 57:4–10.

Huessy, H. R., Metoyer, M., and Townsend, M. 1974. Eight to ten year follow-up of 84 children treated for behavioral disorder in rural Vermont. Acta Paedopsychiatr. 40:230–235.

Huestis, R. D., Arnold, L. E., and Smeltzer, D. J. 1975. Caffeine versus methylphenidate and d-amphetamine in minimal brain dysfunction: A double-blind comparison. Am. J. Psychiatry 132:868–870.

Huey, E. B. 1908. The Psychology and Pedagogy of Reading. MIT Press, Cambridge, Mass. (Reprinted in 1968.)

Hughes, J. R. 1968. Electroencephalography and learning disabilities. In H. R. Myklebust (ed.), Progress in Learning Disabilities, Vol. 1, pp. 113–146. Grune & Stratton, New York.

Hughes, J. R. 1971. Electroencephalography and Learning Disabilities. In H. R. Myklebust (ed.), Progress in Learning Disabilities, Vol. 2, pp. 18–55. Grune & Stratton, New York.

Human Communication and Its Disorders. 1970. NINDS Monograph No. 10.

Humphries, T., Kinsbourne, M., and Swanson, J. 1978. Stimulant effects on cooperation and social interaction between hyperactive children and their mothers. J. Child Psychol. Psychiatry 19:13–22.

Humphries, T., Swanson, J., Kinsbourne, M., and Yiu, L. 1979. Stimulant effects on persistence of motor performance of hyperactive children. J. Pediatr. Psychol. 4:55-66.

Hurwitz, I., Bibace, R. M. A., Wolff, P. H., and Rowbotham, B. M. 1972. The neuropsychological function of normal boys, delinquent boys and boys with learning problems. Percept. Mot. Skills 35:387-394.

Ilg, F., and Ames, L. 1964. School Readiness. Harper & Row, New York.

Illingworth, R. S. 1961. Delayed maturation in development. J. Pediatr. 58:761-770.

Illingworth, R. S. 1963. The clumsy child. In R. MacKeith and M. Bax (eds.), Minimal Cerebral Dysfunction, pp. 26-27. Spastics Society Medical Education and Information Unit in association with William Heinemann Medical Books, Ltd., London.

Illingworth, R. S., and Illingworth, C. M. 1966. Lessons from Childhood. E. & S. Livingstone, London.

Ingram, T. T. S. 1960a. Paediatric aspects of specific developmental dysphasia, dyslexia and dysgraphia. Cerebr. Palsy Bull. 2: 254-277.

Ingram, T. T. S. 1960b. Perceptual disorders causing dyslexia and dysgraphia in cerebral palsy. In Little Club Clinics in Developmental Medicine No. 2, Child Neurology and Cerebral Palsy, pp. 97-104. Spastics Society Medical Education and Information Unit in association with William Heinemann Medical Books, Ltd., London.

Ingram, T. T. S. 1963. Chronic brain syndromes in childhood other than cerebral palsy, epilepsy and mental defect. In R. MacKeith and M. Bax (eds.), Minimal Cerebral Dysfunction, pp. 10-17. Spastics Society Medical Education and Information Unit in association with William Heinemann Medical Books, Ltd., London.

Ingram, T. T. S. 1975. Speech disorders in childhood. In E. H. Lenneberg and E. Lenneberg (eds.), Foundations of Language Development, Vol. 2, pp. 195-261. Academic Press/UNESCO, London.

Ingram, T. T. S., Mason, A. W., and Blackburn, I. 1970. A retrospective study of 82 children with reading disability. Dev. Med. Child Neurol. 12:271-281.

Ingram, T. T. S., and Reid, J. F. 1956. Developmental aphasia observed in a department of child psychiatry. Arch. Dis. Child. 31:161-172.

Jansky, J., and de Hirsch, K. 1972. Preventing Reading Failure. Harper & Row, New York.

Jastak, J. F., Bijou, S. W., and Jastak, S. R. 1965. Wide Range Achievement Test. Guidance Associates, Wilmington, Del.

Jedrysek, E., Klapper, Z., Pope, L., and Wortis, J. 1972. Psychoeducational Evaluation of the Preschool Child. Grune & Stratton, New York.

Jencks, C., et al. 1972. Inequality: A Reassessment of the Effect of Family and Schooling in America. Basic Books, New York.

Jespersen, O. 1956. Growth and Structure of the English Language. Doubleday Anchor Books, New York.

John, E. R., Karmel, B. Z., Corning, W. C., Easton, P., Bown, D., Ahn, H., John, M., Harmony, T., Prichep, L., Toro, A., Gerson, I., Bartlett, F., Thatcher, R., Kaye, H., Valdes, P., and Schwartz, E. 1977. Neurometrics. Science 196:1393–1410.

Johnson, D. J. 1968. The language continuum. Bull. Orton Soc. 18:1–11.

Johnson, D. J., and Myklebust, H. R. 1967. Reading Disabilities: Educational Principles and Practices. Grune & Stratton, New York.

Johnson, R. A., Kenney, J. B., and Davis, J. B. 1976. Developing school policy for use of stimulant drugs for hyperactive children. School Rev. 85:78–96.

Jones, K. L., and Smith, D. W. 1973. Recognition of the fetal alcohol syndrome in early infancy. Lancet 2:999–1001.

Jones, K. L., and Smith, D. W. 1975. The fetal alcohol syndrome. Teratology 12:1–10.

Jones, K. L., Smith, D. W., Streissguth, A. P., and Myrianthopoulos, N. C. 1974. Outcome in offspring of chronic alcoholic women. Lancet 1:1076–1078.

Jordan, T. E. 1964. Early developmental adversity and classroom learning: A prospective inquiry. Am. J. Ment. Defic. 69:360–371.

Juhlin, L., Michaëlsson, G., and Zetterström, O. 1972. Urticaria and asthma induced by food-and-drug additives in patients with aspirin hypersensitivity. J. Allerg. Clin. Immunol. 50:92–98.

Justen, J. E., III, and Harth, R. 1976. The relationship between figure-ground discrimination and color blindness in learning disabled children. J. Learn. Disabil. 9:96–99.

Kahn, D. 1967. The Codebreakers. Macmillan Publishing Co., New York.

Kalverboer, A. F. 1975. A neurobehavioral study in preschool children. Clinics in Developmental Medicine No. 54. Spastics Society Medical Education and Information Unit in association with William Heinemann Medical Books, Ltd., London.

Kalverboer, A. F., Touwen, B. C. L., and Prechtl, H. 1973. Follow-up of infants at risk of minor brain dysfunction. Ann. N.Y. Acad. Sci. 205:173–187.

Kaplan, G. J., Fleshman, J. K., Bender, T. R., Baum, C., and Clark, P. S. 1973. Long-term effects of otitis media: A ten-year cohort study of Alaskan Eskimo children. Pediatrics 52:577–585.

Kappelman, M. M., Kaplan, E., and Ganter, R. L. 1969. A study of learning disorders among disadvantaged children. J. Learn. Disabil. 2:262–268.

Kappelman, M. M., Luck, E., and Ganter, R. L. 1971. Profile of the disadvantaged child with learning disabilities. Am. J. Dis. Child. 121:371–379.

Kappelman, M. M., Rosenstein, A. B., and Ganter, R. L. 1972. Comparison of disadvantaged children with learning disabilities and their successful peer group. Am. J. Dis. Child. 124:875–879.

Kauffman, J. M., and Hallahan, D. P. 1974. The medical model and the science of special education. Except. Child. 41:97–102.

Kaufman, A. S. 1976a. A new approach to the interpretation of test scatter on the WISC-R. J. Learn. Disabil. 9:160–168.

Kaufman, A. S. 1976b. Verbal-performance IQ discrepancies on the WISC-R. J. Consult. Clin. Psychol. 44:739–744.

Kaufman, A. S., and Kaufman, N. L. 1977a. Clinical Evaluation of Young Children with the McCarthy Scales. Grune & Stratton, New York.

Kaufman, A. S., and Kaufman, N. L. 1977b. Research on the McCarthy Scales and its implications for assessment. J. Learn. Disabil. 10:284–291.

Kaufman, N. L., and Kaufman, A. S. 1974. Comparison of normal and minimally brain dysfunctioned children on the McCarthy Scales of children's abilities. J. Clin. Psychol. 30:69–72.

Kavanagh, J. F., and Mattingly, I. G. (eds.). 1972. Language by Ear and by Eye: The Relationships between Speech and Reading. MIT Press, Cambridge, Mass.

Kawi, A. A., and Pasamanick, B. 1958. Association of factors of pregnancy with reading disorders of childhood. JAMA 166:1420–1423.

Kealy, J., and McLeon, J. 1976. Learning disability and socioeconomic status. J. Learn. Disabil. 9:596–599.

Keating, N. R. 1979. A comparison of duration of nystagmus as measured by the Southern California Postrotary Nystagmus Test and electronystagmography. Am. J. Occup. Ther. 33:92–97.

Kender, J. P. 1972. Is there really a WISC profile for poor readers? J. Learn. Disabil. 5:397–400.

Kennard, M. A. 1960. Value of equivocal signs in neurologic diagnosis. Neurology 10:753–764.

Kennard, M. A., Spencer, S., and Fountain, G., Jr. 1941. Hyperactivity in monkeys following lesions of the frontal lobes. J. Neurophysiol. 4:512–524.

Kenny, T. J., and Clemmens, R. L. 1972. Reading problems. Am. Fam. Physician 6:77–80.

Kenny, T. J., Clemmens, R. L., Cicci, R., Lentz, G. A., Jr., Nair, P., and Hudson, B. W. 1972. The medical evaluation of children with reading problems (dyslexia). Pediatrics 49:438–442.

Kenny, T. J., Clemmens, R. L., Hudson, B. W., Lentz, G. A., Jr., Cicci, R., and Nair, P. 1971. Characteristics of children referred because of hyperactivity. J. Pediatr. 79:618–622.

Keogh, B. K. 1973. Perceptual and cognitive styles: Implications for special education. In L. Mann and D. A. Sabatino (eds.), The First Review of Special Education. JSE Press, Philadelphia.

Keogh, B. K. 1974. Optometric vision training programs for children with learning disabilities: Review of issues and research. J. Learn. Disabil. 7:219–231.

Kephart, N. C. 1960. The Slow Learner in the Classroom. Charles E. Merrill Publishing Co., Columbus, Oh.

Kephart, N. C. 1968. Developmental sequences. In S. G. Sapir and A. C. Nitzburg (eds.), 1973, Children with Learning Problems, pp. 318–334. Brunner/Mazel, New York.

Kershner, J. R. 1977. Cerebral dominance in disabled readers, good readers, and gifted children: Search for a valid model. Child Dev. 48:61–67.

Kershner, J. R. 1978. Lateralization in normal 6-year-olds as related to later reading disability. Dev. Psychobiol. 11:309–319.

Keys, M. P. 1977. Dyslexia and reading disorders. In V. C. Kelley (ed.), Practice of Pediatrics, Vol. IV, Part 2, pp. 1–10. Harper & Row, Hagerstown, Md.

Kimura, D. 1967. Functional asymmetry of the brain in dichotic listening. Cortex 3:163-178.

Kimura, D. 1973. The asymmetry of the human brain. Sci. Am. 228(3):70-78.

Kinsbourne, M. 1968. Developmental Gerstmann syndrome. Ped. Clin. North Am. 15:771-778.

Kinsbourne, M. 1973a. Minimal brain dysfunction as a neuro-developmental lag. Ann. N.Y. Acad. Sci. 205:268-273.

Kinsbourne, M. 1973b. School problems. Pediatrics 52:697-710.

Kinsbourne, M. 1975. Cerebral dominance, learning and cognition. In H. R. Myklebust (ed.), Progress in Learning Disabilities, Vol. 3, pp. 201-218. Grune & Stratton, New York.

Kinsbourne, M., and Caplan, P. J. 1979. Children's Learning and Attention Problems. Little, Brown & Co., Boston.

Kinsbourne, M., and Warrington, E. K. 1963a. Developmental factors in reading and writing backwardness. Br. J. Psychol. 54: 145-156.

Kinsbourne, M., and Warrington, E. K. 1963b. The developmental Gerstmann Syndrome. Arch. Neurol. 8:490-501.

Kinsbourne, M., and Warrington, E. K. 1963c. The relevance of delayed acquisition of finger sense to backwardness in reading and writing. In R. MacKeith and M. Bax (eds.), Minimal Cerebral Dysfunction, pp. 62-64. Spastics Society Medical Education and Information Unit in association with William Heinemann Medical Books, Ltd., London.

Kinsbourne, M., and Warrington, E. K. 1963d. A survey of finger sense among retarded readers. In R. MacKeith and M. Bax (eds.), Minimal Cerebral Dysfunction, pp. 65-66. Spastics Society Medical Education and Information Unit in association with William Heinemann Medical Books, Ltd., London.

Kinsbourne, M., and Warrington, E. K. 1964. Disorders of spelling. J. Neurol. Neurosurg. Psychiatry 27:224-228.

Kirk, S. A., and Kirk, W. D. 1978. Uses and abuses of the ITPA. J. Speech Hear. Disord. 43:58-75.

Klapper, Z. S. 1966. Psychoeducational aspects of reading disabilities. Pediatrics 37:366-376.

Klein, P. S., Forbes, G. B., and Nader, P. R. 1975. Effects of starvation in infancy (pyloric stenosis) on subsequent learning abilities. J. Pediatr. 87:8-15.

Kline, C. L., and Lee, N. 1972. A transcultural study of dyslexia: Analysis of language disabilities in 277 Chinese children simultaneously learning to read and write in English and in Chinese. J. Spec. Educ. 6:9-26.

Kline, M. 1974. Why Johnny Can't Add: The Failure of the New Math. Vintage Books, New York.

Klinkerfuss, G. H., Lange, P. H., Weinberg, W. A., and O'Leary, J. 1965. Electroencephalographic abnormalities of children with hyperkinetic behavior. Neurology 15:883-891.

Klonoff, H., and Low, M. 1974. Disordered brain function in young children and early adolescents: Neuropsychological and electroencephalographic correlates. In R. M. Reitan and L. A. Davison (eds.), Clinical Neuropsychology: Current Status and Applications, pp. 121-178. V. H. Winston & Sons, Washington, D.C.

Kluever, R. 1971. Mental abilities and disorders of learning. In H. R. Myklebust (ed.), Progress in Learning Disabilities, Vol. 2, pp. 196-212. Grune & Stratton, New York.

Knights, R. M. 1974. Psychometric assessment of stimulant-induced behavior change. In C. K. Conners (ed.), Clinical Use of Stimulant Drugs in Children, pp. 221-231. Excerpta Medica, Amsterdam.

Knights, R. M., and Bakker, D. J. (eds.). 1976. The Neuropsychology of Learning Disorders: Theoretical Approaches. University Park Press, Baltimore.

Knights, R. M., and Hinton, G. G. 1969. The effects of methylphenidate (Ritalin) on the motor skills and behavior of children with learning problems. J. Nerv. Ment. Dis. 148:643-653.

Knobloch, H., and Pasamanick, B. 1959. Syndrome of minimal cerebral damage in infancy. JAMA 170:1384-1387.

Knobloch, H., and Pasamanick, B. 1966. Prospective studies in the epidemiology of reproductive casualty: Methods, findings, and some implications. Merrill-Palmer Quart. Behav. Dev. 12: 27-43.

Knobloch, H., Rider, R., and Harper, P. 1956. Neuropsychiatric sequelae of prematurity. JAMA 161:581-585.

Kohen-Raz, R. 1970. Developmental patterns of static balance ability and their relation to cognitive school readiness. Pediatrics 46:276-281.

Kohen-Raz, R. 1977. Psychobiological Aspects of Cognitive Growth. Academic Press, New York.

Kohler, I. 1964. The Formation and Transformation of the Perceptual World. In Psychological Issues, Vol. 3, No. 4, Monograph 12, pp. 1-173. International Universities Press, New York.

Kolata, G. B. 1978. Childhood hyperactivity: A new look at treatments and causes. Science 199:515-517.

Kolers, P. A. 1972. Experiments in reading. Sci. Am. 227(1): 84-91.

Kolvin, I., MacKeith, R. C., and Meadow, S. R. (eds.). 1973. Bladder control and Enuresis. Clinics in Developmental Medicine Nos. 48/49. Spastics Society Medical Education and Information Unit in association with William Heinemann Medical Books, Ltd., London.

Koppitz, E. M. 1963. The Bender Gestalt Test for Young Children. Grune & Stratton, New York.

Koppitz, E. M. 1968. Psychological Evaluation of Children's Human Figure Drawings. Grune & Stratton, New York.

Koppitz, E. M. 1971. Children with Learning Disabilities: A Five Year Follow-up Study. Grune & Stratton, New York.

Koppitz, E. M. 1975. The Bender Gestalt Test for Young Children, Vol. 2, Research and Application, pp. 1963-1973. Grune & Stratton, New York.

Koppitz, E. M. 1977. The Visual Aural Digit Span Test. Grune & Stratton, New York.

Kosc, L. 1974. Developmental dyscalculia. J. Learn. Disabil. 7: 164-177.

Kraft, M. B. 1968. Face-hand test. Dev. Med. Child Neurol. 10: 214-219.

Krager, J. M., and Safer, D. M. 1974. Type and prevalence of medication used in the treatment of hyperactive children. N. Engl. J. Med. 291:1118-1120.

Krumboltz, J. D., and Krumboltz, H. B. 1972. Changing Children's Behavior. Prentice-Hall, Englewood Cliffs, N.J.

Kuhlman, F. 1939. Tests of Mental Development. Educational Test Bureau, Minneapolis.

Kurlander, L. F., and Colodny, D. 1969. Psychiatric disability and learning problems. In L. Tarnopol (ed.), Learning Disabilities, pp. 131-153. Charles C Thomas Publishers, Springfield, Ill.

LaBerge, D., and Samuels, S. J. 1977. Basic Processes in Reading: Perception and Comprehension. Lawrence Erlbaum Associates, Hillsdale, N.J.

Lamb, S. H. 1969. The Illinois Test of Psycholinguistic Abilities: Implications for diagnosis and remediation. In L. Tarnopol (ed.), Learning Disabilities, pp. 256–288. Charles C Thomas Publisher, Springfield, Ill.

Landrigan, P. J., Whitworth, R. H., Baloh, R. W., Staehling, N. W., Barthel, W. F., and Rosenblum, B. F. 1975. Neuropsychological dysfunction in children with chronic low-level lead absorption. Lancet 1:708–712.

Larsen, S. C. 1976. The validity of perceptual tests: The debate continues. J. Learn. Disabil. 9:334–337.

Larsen, S. C., Rogers, D., and Sowell, V. 1976. The use of selected perceptual tests in differentiating between normal and learning disabled children. J. Learn. Disabil. 9:85–90.

Lashley, K. S. 1963. Brain Mechanisms and Intelligence. Dover Publications, New York.

Laufer, M. W. 1971. Long-term management and some follow-up findings on the use of drugs with minimal cerebral syndromes. J. Learn. Disabil. 4:519–522.

Laufer, M. W. 1973. Introduction, The hyperkinetic syndrome and minimal brain dysfunction. Pediatr. Ann. 2(5):11–14.

Laufer, M. W. (ed.). 1973. The hyperkinetic syndrome and minimal brain dysfunction. Pediatr. Ann. 2(5).

Laufer, M., and Denhoff, E. 1957. Hyperkinetic behavior syndrome in children. J. Pediatr. 50:463–474.

Laufer, M. W., Denhoff, E., and Rubin, E. Z. 1954. Photo-metrazol activation in children. Electroencephalogr. Clin. Neurophysiol. 6:1–8.

Laufer, M. W., Denhoff, E., and Solomons, G. 1957. Hyperkinetic impulse disorder in children's behavior problems. Psychosom. Med. 19:38–49.

Lawson, L. I. 1965. Language disorders: The relationship of speech defects and reading disabilities. In R. M. Flower, H. F. Gofman and L. I. Lawson (eds.), Reading Disorders: A Multidisciplinary Symposium, pp. 73–80. F. A. Davis Co., Philadelphia.

Lawson, L. J., Jr. 1968. Ophthalmological factors in learning disabilities. In H. R. Myklebust (ed.), Progress in Learning Disabilities, Vol. 1, pp. 147–181. Grune & Stratton, New York.

LD leaders strike back at distorted reporting. 1975. J. Learn. Disabil. 8:316–325.

Lefford, A., Birch, H. G., and Green, G. 1974. The perceptual and cognitive bases for finger localization and selective finger movement in preschool children. Child Dev. 45:335–343.

Lenneberg, E. H. 1964. Language disorders in childhood. Harvard Educ. Rev. 34:152-177.

Lenneberg, E. 1967. Biological Foundations of Language. John Wiley & Sons, New York.

Lenneberg, E. H., and Lenneberg, E. (eds.). 1975. Foundations of Language Development: A Multidisciplinary Approach. 2 Vols. Academic Press, New York.

Lerer, R. J. 1977. Do hyperactive children tend to have abnormal palmar creases? Clin. Pediatr. 7:645-647.

Lerer, R. J., and Lerer, M. P. 1976. The effects of methylphenidate on the soft neurological signs of hyperactive children. Pediatrics 57:521-525.

Lerer, R. J., and Lerer, M. P. 1977. Response of adolescents with minimal brain dysfunction to methylphenidate. J. Learn. Disabil. 10:223-228.

Lerer, R. J., Lerer, M. P., and Artner, J. 1977. The effects of methylphenidate on the handwriting of children with minimal brain dysfunction. J. Pediatr. 91:127-132.

Levin, H., and Williams, J. P. (eds.). 1970. Basic Studies on Reading. Basic Books, New York.

Levy, J., and Levy, J. M. 1978. Human lateralization from head to foot: Sex-related factors. Science 200:1291-1292.

Lewis, C. S. 1961. An Experiment in Criticism. Cambridge University Press, Cambridge, England.

Lewis, R. S., Strauss, A. A., and Lehtinen, L. E. 1960. The Other Child: The Brain-Injured Child. Grune & Stratton, New York.

Lhermitte, M., Deroulsne, J., and Signoret, J. L. 1972. Analyse neuropsychologique du syndrome frontale. [Neuropsychological analysis of the frontal lobe syndrome.] Rev. Neurol. 127: 415-440.

Lindvall, O., and Björklund, A. 1974. The organization of the ascending catecholamine neuron systems in the rat brain as revealed by the glyoxylic acid flourescence method. Acta Physiol. Scand. 412 (suppl.):1-48.

Livingston, R. B., Fulton, J. F., Delgado, J. M. R., Sachs, E., Brendler, S. J., and Davis, G. D. 1947. Stimulation and regional ablation of orbital surface of frontal lobe. Res. Publ. Ass. Nerv. Ment. Dis. 27:405-420.

Lombroso, C., Schwartz, I. H., Clark, D. B., Muench, H., and Barry, J. 1966. Ctenoids in healthy youths. Controlled study of 14- and 6-per-second positive spiking. Neurology 16:1152-1158.

Lucas, A. R., Rodin, E. A., and Simson, C. B. 1965. Neurological assessment of children with early school problems. Dev. Med. Child Neurol. 7:145-156.

Lund, K. A., Foster, G. E., and McCall-Perez, F. C. 1978. The effectiveness of psycholinguistic training: A reevaluation. Except. Child. 44:310-319.

Luria, A. R. 1961. The Role of Speech in the Regulation of Normal and Abnormal Behavior. Liveright Publishing Co., New York.

Luria, A. R. 1963. Restoration of Function after Brain Injury. Macmillan Publishing Co., New York.

Luria, A. R. 1965. Aspects of aphasia. J. Neurol. Sci. 2:278-287.

Luria, A. R. 1973. The Working Brain: An Introduction to Neuropsychology. Basic Books, New York.

Luria, A. R., and Yudovich, F. I. 1971. Speech and the Development of Mental Processes in the Child. Penguin Books, Baltimore.

Lux, J. P. 1977. Detection of learning disabilities using the visually evoked cortical potential. J. Pediatr. Ophthalmol. 14:248-253.

Lycke, E., and Roos, B. F. 1975. Virus infections in infant mice causing persistent impairment of turnover of brain catecholamines. J. Neurol. Sci. 26:49-60.

McCarthy, D. 1972. Manual for the McCarthy Scales of Children's Abilities. Psychological Corporation, New York.

Maccoby, E. E., and Jacklin, C. N. 1974. The Psychology of Sex Differences. Stanford University Press, Stanford, Cal.

McFie, J. 1963. An introduction to the problems of "minimal brain damage." In R. MacKeith and M. Bax (eds.), Minimal Cerebral Dysfunction, pp. 18-23. Spastics Society Medical Education and Information Unit in association with William Heinemann Medical Books, Ltd., London.

McFie, J., and Robertson, J . 1973. Psychological test results of children with thalidomide deformities. Dev. Med. Child Neurol. 15:719-727.

McGaugh, J. L. 1976. Neurobiology and the future of education. School Rev. 85:166-175.

McGlannan, F. K. 1968. Familial characteristics of genetic dyslexia: Preliminary report from a pilot study. J. Learn. Disabil. 1: 185-191.

Mackay, M., Beck, L., and Taylor, R. 1973. Methylphenidate for adolescents with minimal brain dysfunction. N.Y. State J. Med. 73:550-554.

MacKeith, R. 1977. Do disorders of perception occur? Dev. Med. Child Neurol. 19:821–825.

MacKeith, R., and Bax, M. (eds.). 1963. Minimal Cerebral Dysfunction. Clinics in Developmental Medicine No. 10. Spastics Society Medical Education and Information Unit in association with William Heinemann Medical Books, Ltd., London.

Mackworth, J. F. 1972. Some models of the reading process: Learners and skilled readers. In S. G. Sapir and A. C. Nitzburg (eds.), 1973, Children with Learning Problems, pp. 485–516. Brunner/ Mazel, New York.

McMahon, S. A., and Greenberg, L. M. 1977. Serial neurologic examination of hyperactive children. Pediatrics 59:584–587.

Madsen, C. H., Jr., and Madsen, C. K. 1974. Teaching/Discipline: A Positive Approach for Educational Development. Allyn & Bacon, Boston.

Magoun, H. W. 1963. The Waking Brain. Charles C Thomas Publisher, Springfield, Ill.

Maire, F. W., and Patton, H. D. 1954. Hyperactivity and pulmonary edema from rostral hypothalamic lesions in rats. Am. J. Physiol. 178:315–320.

Makita, K. 1968. The rarity of reading disability in Japanese children. Am. J. Orthopsychiatry 38:599–614.

Mann, L. 1970. Perceptual training: Misdirections and redirections. Am. J. Orthopsychiatry 40:30–38.

Mann, L. 1971a. Perceptual training revisited: The training of nothing at all. Rehabil. Lit. 32:322–327, 335.

Mann, L. 1971b. Psychometric Phrenology. J. Spec. Educ. 5:3–14.

Mann, L. 1972. Frostig Developmental Tests of Visual Perception. In O. K. Buros (ed.), Seventh Mental Measurements Yearbook, Vol. 2, pp. 1272–1276. Gryphon Press, Highland Park, N.J.

Mann, L., and Goodman, L. 1976. Perceptual training: A critical retrospect. In E. Schopler and R. J. Reichler (eds.), Psychopathology and Child Development, pp. 271–289. Plenum Press, New York.

Mann, L., and Phillips, W. A. 1967. Fractional practices in special education: A critique. Except. Child. 33:311–317.

Margolin, J. B., Roman, M., and Harari, C. 1955. Reading disability in the delinquent child: A microcosm of psychosocial pathology. Am. J. Orthopsychiatry 25:25–35.

Martinius, J. W., and Hoovey, Z. B. 1972. Bilateral synchrony of occipital alpha waves, oculomotor activity and "attention" in children. Electroencephalogr. Clin. Neurophysiol. 32:349–356.

Masland, R. L., and Cratty, B. J. 1972. The nature of the reading process, the rationale of non-educational remedial methods. In E. O. Calkins (ed.), Reading Forum, pp. 141–175. DHEW Publication No. (NIH) 72-44.

Mason, A. 1967. Specific (developmental) dyslexia. Dev. Med. Child Neurol. 9:183–190.

Masters, L., and Marsh, G. E., II. 1978. Middle ear pathology as a factor in learning disabilities. J. Learn. Disabil. 11:103–106.

Matheny, A. P., Dolan, A. B., and Wilson, R. S. 1976. Twins with academic learning problems: Antecedent characteristics. Am. J. Orthopsychiatry 46:464–469.

Matkin, N. D. 1968. The child with a marked high-frequency hearing impairment. Pediatr. Clin. North Am. 15:677–690.

Mattingly, I. G. 1972. Reading, the linguistic process, and linguistic awareness. In J. F. Kavanagh and I. G. Mattingly (eds.), Language by Ear and by Eye, pp. 133–147. MIT Press, Cambridge, Mass.

Mattis, S., French, J. H., and Rapin, I. 1975. Dyslexia in children and young adults: Three independent neuropsychological syndromes. Dev. Med. Child Neurol. 17:150–163.

Mattson, R. H., and Calverly, J. R. 1968. Dextroamphetamine sulfate induced dyskinesias. JAMA 204:400–402.

Mauser, A. J. 1977. Assessing the Learning Disabled: Selected Instruments. Academic Therapy Publications, San Rafael, Cal.

May, C. D. 1975. Food allergy: A commentary. Pediatr. Clin. North Am. 22:217–220.

Mayron, L. W. 1979. Allergy, learning, and behavior problems. J. Learn. Disabil. 12:32–42.

Mednick, B. R. 1977. Intellectual and behavioral functioning of ten- to twelve-year-old children who showed certain transient symptoms in the neonatal period. Child Dev. 48:844–853.

Meier, J. H. 1971. Prevalence and characteristics of learning disabilities found in second grade children. J. Learn. Disabil. 4:1–16.

Meier, M. J. 1974. Some challenge for clinical neuropsychology. In R. M. Reitan and L. A. Davison (eds.), Clinical Neuropsychology, pp. 289–323. V. H. Winston & Sons, Washington, D.C.

Melton, D. 1975. Burn the Schools—Save the Children. Thomas Y. Crowell, New York.

Mendelson, W., Johnson, N., and Stewart, M. A. 1971. Hyperactive children as teenagers: A follow-up study. J. Nerv. Ment. Dis. 153:273–279.

Menkes, J. H. 1977. Early feeding history of children with learning disorders. Dev. Med. Child Neurol. 19:169–171.

Menkes, J. H., and Schain, R. J. (eds.). 1971. Learning Disorders in Children. Ross Conference on Pediatric Research No. 61. Ross Laboratories, Columbus, Oh.

Menkes, J. H., Welcher, D. W., Levi, H. S., Dallas, J., and Gretsky, N. E. 1972. Relationship of elevated blood tyrosine to the ultimate intellectual performance of premature infants. Pediatrics 49:218–224.

Menkes, M., Rowe, J., and Menkes, J. 1967. A 25-year follow-up study on the hyperkinetic child with minimal brain dysfunction. Pediatrics 39:393–399.

Merklein, R. A., and Briskey, R. J. 1962. Audiometric findings in children referred to a program for language disorders. Volta Rev. 64:294–298.

Mettler, F. A., and Mettler, C. C. 1942. The effects of striatal injury. Brain 65:242–255.

Miller, G. A. 1956. The magical number seven, plus or minus two: Some limits on our capacity for processing information. Psychol. Rev. 63:81–97.

Miller, J. S. 1978. Hyperactive children: A ten-year study. Pediatrics 61:217–223.

Miller, R. G., Jr., Palkes, H. S., and Stewart, M. A. 1973. Hyperactive children in suburban elementary schools. Child Psychiatry Hum. Dev. 4:121–127.

Millichap, J. G. 1973. Drugs in management of minimal brain dysfunction. Ann. N.Y. Acad. Sci. 205:321–334.

Millichap, J. G. 1978. Growth of hyperactive children treated with methylphenidate. J. Learn. Disabil. 9:567–570.

Millichap, J. G., Aymot, F., Sturgis, L. H., Larsen, K. W., and Egan, R. A. 1968. Hyperkinetic behavior and learning disorders. III. Battery of neuropsychological tests in controlled trial of methylphenidate. Am. J. Dis. Child. 116:235–244.

Millichap, J. G., Egan, R. W., Hart, W. H., and Sturgis, L. H. 1969. Auditory perceptual deficit correlated with EEG dysrhythmias. Response to diphenylhydantoin sodium. Neurology 19:870–872.

Millichap, J. G., and Fowler, G. W. 1967. Treatment of "minimal brain dysfunction" syndrome. Pediatr. Clin. North Am. 14:767–777.

Millichap, J. G., and Johnson, F. H. 1974. Methylphenidate in hyperkinetic behavior: Relation of response to degree of activity and brain damage. In C. K. Conners (ed.), Clinical Use of Stimulant Drugs in Children, pp. 130–140. Excerpta Medica, Amsterdam.

Minde, K., Lewin, D., Weiss, G., Lavigueur, H., Douglas, V., and Sykes, E. 1971. The hyperactive child in elementary school: A five-year controlled follow-up. Except. Child. 38:215–221.

Minde, K., Webb, G., and Sykes, D. 1968. Studies on the hyperactive child. VI. Prenatal and paranatal factors associated with hyperactivity. Dev. Med. Child Neurol. 10:355–363.

Minde, K., Weiss, G., and Mendelson, N. 1972. A 5-year follow-up study of 91 hyperactive school children. J. Am. Acad. Child Psychiatry 11:595–610.

Minskoff, J. G. 1973. Differential approaches to prevalence estimates of learning disabilities. Ann. N.Y. Acad. Sci. 205:139–145.

Money, J. 1962a. Dyslexia: A postconference review. In J. Money (ed.), Reading Disability: Progress and Research Needs in Dyslexia, pp. 9–33. Johns Hopkins Press, Baltimore.

Money, J. (ed.). 1962b. Reading Disability: Progress and Research Needs in Dyslexia. Johns Hopkins Press, Baltimore.

Money, J. (ed.). 1966a. The Disabled Reader: Education of the Dyslexic Child. Johns Hopkins Press, Baltimore.

Money, J. 1966b. On learning and not learning to read. In J. Money (ed.), The Disabled Reader: Education of the Dyslexic Child, pp. 21–40. Johns Hopkins Press, Baltimore.

Money, J., and Alexander, D. 1966. Turner's syndrome: Further demonstration of the presence of specific cognitional deficits. J. Med. Genet. 3:47–48.

Monroe, M. 1932. Children Who Cannot Read. University of Chicago Press, Chicago.

Montagu, J. D. 1975. The hyperkinetic child: A behavioural, electrodermal and EEG investigation. Dev. Med. Child Neurol. 17:299–305.

Montagu, J. D., and Swarbrick, L. 1975. Effect of amphetamines in hyperkinetic children: Stimulant or sedative? A pilot study. Dev. Med. Child Neurol. 17:293–298.

Montessori, M. 1971. The Montessori Method. Schocken Books, New York.

Montessori, M. 1972. The Discovery of the Child. Ballantine Books, New York.

Morrison, F. J., Giordani, B., and Nagy, J. 1977. Reading disability: An information-processing analysis. Science 196:77–79.

Morrison, J. R., and Stewart, M. A. 1971. A family study of the hyperactive child syndrome. Biol. Psychiatry 3:189–195.

Morrison, J., and Stewart, M. 1973. The psychiatric status of the legal families of adopted hyperactive children. Arch. Gen. Psychiatry 28:888–891.

Morrison, J. R., and Stewart, M. A. 1974. Bilateral inheritance as evidence for polygenicity in the hyperactive child syndrome. J. Nerv. Ment. Dis. 158:226–228.

Moskowitz, M. A., and Wurtman, R. J. 1975. Catecholamines and neurologic diseases. N. Engl. J. Med. 293:274–280, 332–338.

Mottram, V. H. 1952. The Physical Basis of Personality. Penguin Books, Baltimore.

Mountcastle, V. B. (ed.). 1962. Interhemispheric Relations and Cerebral Dominance. Johns Hopkins Press, Baltimore.

Muehl, S., and Forell, E. R. 1973. A followup study of disabled readers: Variables related to high school reading performance. Read. Res. Quart. 8:110–123.

Muehl, S., Knott, J., and Benton, A. L. 1965. EEG abnormality and psychological test performance in reading disability. Cortex 1:434–440.

Muzyczka, M. J., and Erickson, M. T. 1976. WISC characteristics of reading disabled children identified by three objective methods. Percept. Mot. Skills 43:595–602.

Myklebust, H. R. (ed.). 1968. Progress in Learning Disabilities, Vol. 1. Grune & Stratton, New York.

Myklebust, H. R. 1973. Identification and diagnosis of children with learning disabilities: An interdisciplinary study of criteria. In S. Walzer and P. H. Wolff (eds.), Minimal Cerebral Dysfunction in Children, pp. 55–77. Grune & Stratton, New York.

Natchez, G. (ed.). 1968. Children with Reading Problems. Basic Books, New York.

Needleman, H. L. 1973. Lead poisoning in children: Neurologic implications of widespread subclinical intoxication. In S. Walzer and P. H. Wolff (eds.), Minimal Cerebral Dysfunction in Children, pp. 47–54. Grune & Stratton, New York.

Needleman, H. L., Gunnoe, C., Leviton, A., Reed, R., Peresie, H., Moher, C., and Barrett, B. S. 1979. Deficits in psychologic and classroom performance of children with elevated dentine lead levels. N. Engl. J. Med. 300:689–695.

Neisser, U. 1967. Cognitive Psychology. Appleton-Century-Crofts, New York.

Neligan, G. A., Kolvin, I., Scott, D. Mcl., and Garside, R. F. 1976. Born Too Soon or Born Too Small. Clinics in Developmental Medicine No. 61. Spastics Society Medical Education and Information Unit in association with William Heinemann Medical Books, Ltd., London.

Newbrough, J. R., and Kelly, J. G. 1962. A study of reading achievement in a population of school children. In J. Money (ed.), Reading Disability: Progress and Research Needs in Dyslexia, pp. 61–72. Johns Hopkins Press, Baltimore.

Newcomer, P. L., and Goodman, L. 1975. Effect of modality of instruction on the learning of meaningful and nonmeaningful material by auditory and visual learners. J. Spec. Educ. 9:261–269.

Newton, J. 1976. Minimal brain dysfunction: Toward an understanding between school and physician. JAMA 235:2524–2525.

Newton, J. (ed.). 1978. A Multidisciplinary Approach to Learning Disability. American School Health Association, Kent, Oh.

Nichamin, S. J. 1972. Recognizing minimal cerebral dysfunction in the infant and toddler. Clin. Pediatr. 11:255–257.

Njiokiktjien, C. J., Visser, S. L., and deRijke, W. 1977. EEG and visual evoked responses in children with learning disorders. Neuropädiatrie 8:134–147.

Norn, M. S., Rindzuinski, E., and Skyvsgaard, H. 1969. Ophthalmologic and orthoptic examinations of dyslexics. Acta Ophthalmol. 47:147–160.

Norton, S., Mullenix, P., and Culver, B. 1976. Comparison of the structure of hyperactive behavior in rats after brain damage from X-irradiation, carbon monoxide and pallidal lesions. Brain Res. 116:49–67.

Novak, H. S., Bonaventura, E., and Merenda, P. F. 1973. A scale for early detection of children with learning problems. Except. Child. 40:98–105.

Oakland, T. (ed.). 1977. Psychological and Educational Assessment of Minority Children. Brunner/Mazel, New York.

Oettinger, L., Gauch, R. R., and Majovski, L. V. 1977. Maturity and growth in children with MBD. In J. G. Millichap (ed.),

Learning Disabilities and Related Disorders, pp. 141-149. Year Book Medical Publishers, Chicago.

Oettinger, L., Majovski, L. V., Limbeck, G. A., and Gauch, R. 1974. Bone age in children with minimal brain dysfunction. Percept. Mot. Skills 39:1127-1131.

Ohlrich, E. S., and Barnet, A. B. 1972. Auditory-evoked responses during the first year of life. Electroencephalogr. Clin. Neurophysiol. 32:161-169.

Olds, J. 1962. Hypothalamic substrates of reward. Physiol. Rev. 42:554-604.

O'Leary, K. D., Pelham, W. E., Rosenbaum, A., and Price, G. H. 1976. Behavioral treatment of hyperkinetic children: An experimental analysis of its usefulness. Clin. Pediatr. 15:510-515.

O'Leary, S. G., and Pelham, W. E. 1978. Behavior therapy and withdrawal of stimulant medication in hyperactive children. Pediatrics 61:211-217.

Olson, A. V. 1968. Factor analytic studies of the Frostig Developmental Test of Visual Perception. J. Spec. Educ. 2:429-433.

Olson, M. E. 1975. Minimal cerebral dysfunction: The child referred for school-related problems. Pediatr. Ann. 4:467-478.

Olton, D. S. 1977. Spatial memory. Sci. Am. 236(6):82-98.

O'Malley, J. E., and Eisenberg, L. 1973. The hyperkinetic syndrome. In S. Walzer and P. H. Wolff (eds.), Minimal Cerebral Dysfunction in Children, pp. 95-103. Grune & Stratton, New York.

Omenn, G. S. 1973. Genetic issues in the syndrome of minimal brain dysfunction. In S. Walzer and P. H. Wolff (eds.), Minimal Cerebral Dysfunction in Children, pp. 5-17. Grune & Stratton, New York.

Orton, J. L. 1966. The Orton-Gillingham approach. In J. Money (ed.), The Disabled Reader: Education of the Dyslexic Child, pp. 119-145. Johns Hopkins Press, Baltimore.

Orton, S. 1928. An impediment to learning to read—A neurological explanation of the reading disability. School Soc. 28:286-290.

Orton, S. T. 1937. Reading, Writing and Speech Problems in Children. W. W. Norton Co., New York.

Orton, S. T. 1966. "Word-Blindness" in School Children and Other Papers on Strephosymbolia (Specific Language Disability—Dyslexia), 1925-1946. J. L. Orton (ed.), The Orton Society, Monograph No. 2. Pomfret, Conn.

Osterreith, P. A. 1944. Le test de copie d'une figure complexe. Arch. Psychol. 30:205–356.

Ott, J. N. 1976. Influence of flourescent lights on hyperactivity and learning disabilities. J. Learn. Disabil. 9:417–422.

Ottenbacher, K. 1978. Identifying vestibular processing dysfunction in learning disabled children. Am. J. Occup. Ther. 32:217–221.

Owen, F. W., Adams, P. A., Forrest, T., Stolz, L. M., and Fisher, S. 1971. Learning Disorders in Children: Sibling Studies. Monogr. Soc. Res. Child Dev. (serial no. 144). pp. 1–77.

Ozer, M. N. 1968. The neurological evaluation of school-age children. J. Learn. Disabil. 1:84–87.

Page, J. G., Bernstein, J. E., Janicki, R. S., and Michelli, F. A. 1974. A multi-clinic trial of pemoline in childhood hyperkinesis. In C. K. Conners (ed.), Clinical Use of Stimulant Drugs in Children, pp. 98–124. Excerpta Medica, Amsterdam.

Page-El, E., and Grossman, H. J. 1973. Neurological appraisal in learning disorders. Pediatr. Clin. North Am. 20:599–605.

Paine, R. S. 1962. Minimal chronic brain syndromes in children. Dev. Med. Child Neurol. 4:21–27.

Paine, R. S. 1968. Syndromes of "minimal cerebral damage." Pediatr. Clin. North Am. 15:779–801.

Paine, R. S., and Oppé, T. E. 1966. Neurological Examination of Children. Clinics in Developmental Medicine No. 20/21. Spastics Society Medical Education and Information Unit in association with William Heinemann Medical Books, Ltd., London.

Palmer, S. 1978. Minimal brain dysfunction. In S. Palmer and S. Ekvall (eds.), Pediatric Nutrition in Developmental Disorders, pp. 73–80. Charles C Thomas Publisher, Springfield, Ill.

Palmer, S., Rapoport, J. L., and Quinn, P. O. 1975. Food additives and hyperactivity. Clin. Pediatr. 14:956–959.

Paraskevopoulos, J. N., and Kirk, S. A. 1969. The Development and Psychometric Characteristics of the Revised Illinois Test of Psycholinguistic Abilities. University of Illinois Press, Urbana, Ill.

Park, G. E., and Schneider, K. A. 1975. Thyroid function in relation to dyslexia (reading failures). J. Read. Behav. 7:197–199.

Park, R. 1978. Performance on geometric figure copying tests as predictors of types of errors in decoding. Read. Res. Quart. 14:100–118.

Parmenter, C. L. 1975. The asymmetrical tonic neck reflex in normal first and third grade children. Am. J. Occup. Ther. 29:463–468.

Paternite, C. E., Loney, J., and Langhorne, J. E. 1976. Relationship between symptomatology and SES-related factors in hyperkinetic/MBD boys. Am. J. Orthopsychiatry 46:291–301.

Patten, B. M. 1973. Visually mediated thinking: A report of the case of Albert Einstein. J. Learn. Disabil. 6:415–420.

Patterson, G. R. 1975. Families. Research Press, Campaign, Ill.

Patterson, G. R., and Gullion, M. E. 1971. Living with Children: New Methods for Parents and Teachers. Research Press, Champaign, Ill.

Pauling, L. 1970. Vitamin C and the Common Cold. W. H. Freeman & Co., San Francisco.

Penfield, W., and Roberts, L. 1959. Speech and Brain Mechanisms. Princeton University Press, Princeton.

Peters, J. E., Davis, J. S., Goolsby, C. M., Clements, S. D., and Hicks, T. J. 1973. Physician's Handbook: Screening for MBD. CIBA, Summit, N.J.

Peters, J. E., Dykman, R. A., Ackerman, P. T., and Romine, J. S. 1974. The special neurological examination. In C. K. Conners (ed.), Clinical Use of Stimulant Drugs in Children, pp. 53–66. Excerpta Medica, Amsterdam.

Peters, J. E., Romine, J. S., and Dykman, R. A. 1975. A special neurologic examination of children with learning disabilities. Dev. Med. Child Neurol. 17:63–78.

Pharmacotherapy of Children. 1973. Psychopharmacol. Bull. (special issue). DHEW Publication No. (HSM) 73-9002.

Phillips, J. L. 1969. The Origins of Intellect: Piaget's Theory. W. H. Freeman & Co., San Francisco.

Piaget, J. 1969. The Mechanisms of Perception. Basic Books, New York.

Piaget, J. 1970. Science of Education and the Psychology of the Child. Viking Press, New York.

Piaget, J., Inhelder, B., and Szeminska, A. 1960. The Child's Conception of Geometry. Basic Books, New York.

Pièron, H. 1945. La Sensation, Guide de Vie. [Sensation, the Guide to Life.] Gallimard, Paris.

Pincus, J. H., and Tucker, G. 1974. Behavioral Neurology. Oxford University Press, New York.

Poremba, C. P. 1975. Learning disabilities, youth and delin-
quency: Programs for intervention. In H. R. Myklebust (ed.),
Progress in Learning Disabilities, Vol. 3, pp. 123–149. Grune &
Stratton, New York.

Porges, S. W., Walter, G. F., Korb, R. J., and Sprague, R. L. 1975.
The influences of methylphenidate on heart rate and behavioral
measures of attention in hyperactive children. Child Dev. 46:
727–733.

Postman, N., and Weingartner, C. 1971. The Soft Revolution. Del-
acorte Press, New York.

Prechtl, H. 1960. The long-term value of the neurological examination of the newborn infant. Dev. Med. Child Neurol. 2:69–74.

Prechtl, H. F. R. 1961. Neurological sequelae of prenatal and paranatal complications. In B. M. Foss (ed.), Determinants of Infant
Behavior, pp. 45–48. John Wiley & Sons, New York.

Prechtl, H. F. R. 1962. Reading difficulties as a neurological problem in childhood. In J. Money (ed.), Reading Disability: Progress and Research Needs in Dyslexia, pp. 187–193. Johns Hopkins Press, Baltimore.

Prechtl, H. F. R. 1963. The mother-child interaction in babies with
minimal brain damage (a follow-up study). In B. M. Foss (ed.),
Determinants of Infant Behaviour, Vol. 2, pp. 53–66. John
Wiley & Sons, New York.

Prechtl, H. F. R. 1965. Prognostic value of neurological signs in
the newborn infant. Proc. Roy. Soc. Med. 58:3–4.

Prechtl, H., and Beintema, D. 1964. The neurological examination
of the full term newborn infant. Clinics in Developmental Medicine No. 12. Spastics Society Medical Education and Information Unit in association with William Heinemann Medical
Books, Ltd., London.

Prechtl, H. F. R., and Stemmer, C. J. 1962. The choreiform syndrome in children. Dev. Med. Child Neurol. 4:119–127.

Preston, M. S., Guthrie, J. T., and Childs, B. 1974. Visual evoked
responses (VERs) in normal and disabled readers. Psychophysiology 11:452–457.

Preston, M. S., Guthrie, J. T., Kirsch, I., Gertman, D., and Childs,
B. 1977. VERs in normal and disabled adult readers. Psychophysiology 14:8–14.

Pribram, K. H. 1969. The neuropsychology of remembering. Sci.
Am. 220(1):73–86.

Pricher, L. S., Sutton, S., and Hakerem, G. 1976. Evoked potentials in hyperkinetic and normal children. Psychophysiology 13: 419–428.

Prout, H. T. 1977. Behavioral intervention with hyperactive children: A review. J. Learn. Disabil. 10:141–146.

Quinn, P. O., and Rapoport, J. L. 1974. Minor physical anomalies and neurologic status in hyperactive boys. Pediatrics 53:742–747.

Quinn, P. O., and Rapoport, J. L. 1975. One-year follow-up of hyperactive boys treated with imipramine or methylphenidate. Am. J. Psychiatry 132:241–245.

Quinn, P. O., Renfield, M., Burg, C., and Rapoport, J. L. 1977. Minor physical anomalies: A newborn screening and one-year follow-up. J. Am. Acad. Child Psychiatry 16:662–669.

Rabinovitch, R. D. 1962. Dyslexia: Psychiatric considerations. In J. Money (ed.), Reading Disability: Progress and Research Needs in Dyslexia, pp. 73–79. Johns Hopkins Press, Baltimore.

Rabinovitch, R., Drew, A., DeJong, R., Ingram, W., and Withey, L. 1956. A research approach to reading retardation. Proc. Assoc. Res. Nerv. Ment. Disord. 34:363–396.

Rabinovitch, R. D., and Ingram, W. 1962. Neuropsychiatric considerations in reading retardation. Read. Teacher 15:433–438.

Rapin, I. 1974. Hypoactive labyrinths and motor development. Clin. Pediatr. 13:922–937.

Rapoport, J. L., and Benoit, M. 1975. The relation of direct home observations to the clinic evaluation of hyperactive school age boys. J. Child Psychol. Psychiatry 16:141–147.

Rapoport, J. L., Buchsbaum, M. S., Zahn, T. P., Weingartner, H., Ludlow, C., and Mikkelsen, E. J. 1978. Dextroamphetamine: Cognitive and behavioral effects in normal prepubertal boys. Science 199:560–563.

Rapoport, J. L., Pandoni, C., Renfield, M., Lake, C. R., and Ziegler, M. G. 1977. Newborn dopamine-β-hydroxylase, minor physical anomalies, and infant temperament. Am. J. Psychiatry 134: 676–679.

Rapoport, J. L., Quinn, P. O., and Lamprecht, F. 1974. Minor physical anomalies and plasma dopamine-beta-hydroxylase in hyperactive boys. Am. J. Psychiatry 131:386–390.

Rawson, M. B. 1968. Developmental Language Disability. Johns Hopkins Press, Baltimore.

Reed, H. B. C., Jr. 1979. Biological defects and special education—An issue in personnel preparation. J. Spec. Educ. 13:9–33.

Reimer, D. C., Eaves, L. C., Richards, R., and Crichton, J. U. 1975. Name-printing as a test of developmental maturity. Dev. Med. Child Neurol. 17:486–492.

Reitan, R. M. 1966. A research program on the psychological effects of brain lesions in human beings. In N. R. Ellis (ed.), International Review of Research in Mental Retardation, pp. 153–218. Academic Press, New York.

Reitan, R. M., and Boll, T. J. 1973. Neuropsychological correlates of minimal brain dysfunction. Ann. N.Y. Acad. Sci. 205:65–88.

Reitan, R. M., and Davison, L. A. (eds.). 1974. Clinical Neuropsychology: Current Status and Applications. V. H. Winston & Sons, Washington, D.C.

Renfrew, C., and Murphy, K. (eds.). 1964. The Child Who Does Not Talk. Clinics in Developmental Medicine No. 13. Spastics Society Medical Education and Information Unit in association with William Heinemann Medical Books, Ltd., London.

Resnick, D. P., and Resnick, L. B. 1977. The nature of literacy: An historical exploration. Harvard Educ. Rev. 47:370–385.

Reuben, R. N., and Bakwin, H. 1968. Developmental clumsiness. Pediatr. Clin. North Am. 15:601–610.

Rey, A. 1959. Test de Copie et de Reproduction de Mémoire de Figures Géometriques Complexes: Manuel. [Test Manual: Geometric figures for copying and reproduction from memory.] Les Editions du Centre de Psychologie Appliquée, Paris.

Richardson, S. A., Birch, H. G., and Hertzig, M. E. 1973. School performance of children who were severely malnourished in infancy. Am. J. Ment. Defic. 77:623–632.

Rie, H. E. 1975. Hyperactivity in children. Am. J. Dis. Child. 129:783–789.

Rie, H. E., Rie, E. D., Stewart, S., and Ambuel, J. P. 1976. Effects of Ritalin on underachieving children: A replication. Am. J. Orthopsychiatry 46:313–322.

Ringler, L. H., and Smith, I. L. 1973. Learning modality and word recognition of first-grade children. J. Learn. Disabil. 6:307–312.

Robbins, M. P., and Glass, G. 1968. The Doman-Delacato rationale: A critical analysis. In J. Hellmuth (ed.), Educational Therapy. Special Child Publications, Vol. 2, pp. 321–377, Seattle.

Robinson, H. M., and Smith, H. K. 1962. Reading clinic clients—

Ten years after. Read. Clin. 63:22–27.

Robinson, M. E., and Schwartz, L. B. 1973. Visuo-motor skills and reading ability: A longitudinal study. Dev. Med. Child Neurol. 15:281–286.

Roche, A. F., Lipman, R. S., Overall, J. E., and Hung, W. 1979. The effects of stimulant medications on the growth of hyperkinetic children. Pediatrics 63:847–850.

Rodgers, B. 1978. Feeding in infancy and later ability and attainment: A longitudinal study. Dev. Med. Child Neurol. 20:421–426.

Rogers, P. T., Accardo, P., Capute, A. J., and Maguire, M. Young Adulthood Accomplishments of the Child with Minimal Cerebral Dysfunction: A Ten-Year Follow-up Study. In preparation.

Rogers, W. B., Jr., and Rogers, R. A. 1972. A new simplified preschool readiness experimental screening scale. Clin. Pediatr. 11:558–562.

Rohn, R. D., Sarles, R. M., Kenny, T. J., Reynolds, B. J., and Heald, F. P. 1977. Adolescents who attempt suicide. J. Pediatr. 90:636–638.

Rosenberg, J. B., and Weller, G. M. 1973. Minor physical anomalies and academic performance in young school children. Dev. Med. Child Neurol. 15:131–135.

Rosenthal, R., and Jacobson, L. F. 1968. Teacher expectations for the disadvantaged. Sci. Am. 218(4):19–23.

Ross, D. M., and Ross, S. A. 1976. Hyperactivity: Research, Theory, Action. John Wiley & Sons, New York.

Rossi, A. O. 1967. Psychoneurologically impaired child. N.Y. State J. Med. 67:902–912.

Roucek, J. S. (ed.). 1965. Programmed Teaching: A Symposium on Automation in Education. Philosophical Library, New York.

Roucek, J. S. (ed.). 1969. The Slow Learner. Philosophical Library, New York.

Rourke, B. P. 1975. Brain-behaviour relationships in children with learning disabilities: A research programme. Am. Psychol. 30:911–920.

Rourke, B. P., Dietrich, M., and Young, I. C. 1973. Significance of WISC verbal-performance discrepancies for younger children with learning disabilities. Percept. Mot. Skills 36:275–282.

Routtenberg, A. 1978. The reward system of the brain. Sci. Am. 239(5):154–164.

Rozin, P., Poritsky, S., and Sotsky, R. 1971. American children with reading problems can easily learn to read English represented by Chinese characters. Science 171:1264-1267.

Rubin, E. Z., and Braun, J. S. 1968. Behavioral and learning disabilities associated with cognitive-motor dysfunction. Percept. Mot. Skills 26:171-180.

Rubin, R. A., Rosenblatt, C., and Balow, B. 1973. Psychological and educational sequelae of prematurity. Pediatrics 52:352-363.

Ruch, T. C., and Shenkin, H. A. 1943. The relation of area 13 on orbital surface of frontal lobes to hyperactivity and hyperphagia in monkeys. J. Neurophysiol. 6:349-360.

Rudel, R. G., and Denckla, M. B. 1974. Relation of forward and backward digit repetition to neurological impairment in children with learning disabilities. Neuropsychologia 12:109-118.

Rudel, R. G., and Denckla, M. B. 1976. Relationship of IQ and reading score to visual, spatial, and temporal matching tasks. J. Learn. Disabil. 9:169-178.

Rudel, R. G., Teuber, H. L., and Twitchell, T. E. 1974. Levels of impairment of sensori-motor functions in children with early brain damage. Neuropsychologia 12:95-108.

Rugel, R. P. 1974. WISC subtest scores of disabled readers: A review with respect to Bannatyne's recategorization. J. Learn. Disabil. 7:48-56.

Rutter, M. 1969. The concept of dyslexia. In P. Wolff and R. Mac-Keith (eds.), Planning for Better Learning, pp. 129-139. Spastics Society Medical Education and Information Unit in association with William Heinemann Medical Books, Ltd., London.

Rutter, M. 1972. The effects of language delay on development. In M. Rutter and J. A. M. Martin (eds.), The Child with Delayed Speech, pp. 176-188. Spastics Society Medical Education and Information Unit in association with William Heinemann Medical Books, Ltd., London.

Rutter, M. 1974. Emotional disorder and educational underachievement. Arch. Dis. Child. 49:249-256.

Rutter, M. 1977. Brain damage syndromes in childhood: Concepts and findings. J. Child Psychol. Psychiatry 18:1-21.

Rutter, M., Graham, P., and Birch, H. G. 1966. Interrelations between the choreiform syndrome, reading disability and psychiatric disorder in children of 8-11 years. Dev. Med. Child Neurol. 8:149-159.

Rutter, M., and Martin, J. A. M. (eds.). 1972. The Child with Delayed Speech. Clinics in Developmental Medicine No. 43. Spastics Society Medical Education and Information Unit in association with William Heinemann Medical Books, Ltd., London.

Rutter, M., Tizard, J., Yule, W., Graham, P., and Whitmore, K. 1976. Isle of Wight studies, 1964–1974. Psychol. Med. 6:313–332.

Rutter, M., and Yule, W. 1975. The concept of specific reading retardation. J. Child Psychol. Psychiatry 16:181–197.

Sabatino, D. A. 1979. Ability or Process Training: Rumplestiltskin Revisited. Paper presented at "The Spectrum of Developmental Disabilities in the Preschool Child," March 20, Baltimore.

Sabatino, D. A., Abbott, J. C., and Becker, J. T. 1974. What does the Frostig DTVP measure? Except. Child. 40:453–454.

Sabatino, D. A., and Dorfman, N. 1974. Matching learner aptitude to two commercial reading programs. Except. Child. 41:85–90.

Sabatino, D. A., Ysseldyke, J. E., and Woolston, J. 1973. Diagnostic-prescriptive perceptual training with mentally retarded children. Am. J. Ment. Defic. 78:7–14.

Safer, D. J. 1973. A familial factor in minimal brain dysfunction. Behav. Genet. 3:175–186.

Safer, D. J., and Allen, R. P. 1973. Factors influencing the suppressant effects of two stimulant drugs on the growth of hyperactive children. Pediatrics 51:660–667.

Safer, D. J., and Allen, R. P. 1976. Hyperactive Children: Diagnosis and Management. University Park Press, Baltimore.

Safer, D., Allen, R., and Barr, E. 1972. Depression of growth in hyperactive children on stimulant drugs. N. Engl. J. Med. 287:217–220.

Safer, D. J., Allen, R. P., and Barr, E. 1975. Growth rebound after termination of stimulant drugs. J. Pediatr. 86:113–116.

Saffran, E. M., and Marin, O. S. 1977. Reading without phonology: Evidence from aphasia. Quart. J. Exp. Psychol. 29:515–525.

Sakamoto, T., and Makita, K., 1973. Japan. In J. Downing (ed.), Comparative Reading, pp. 440–465. Macmillan Publishing Co., New York.

Salk, L. 1973. Emotional factors in pediatric practice. In M. W. Laufer (ed.), The hyperkinetic syndrome and minimal brain dysfunction. Pediatr. Ann. 2(5):83–86.

Sapir, S. G. 1966. Sex differences in perceptual motor development. Percept. Mot. Skills 22:987-992.

Sapir, S. G. 1971. Learning disability and deficit centered classroom training. In J. Hellmuth (ed.), Cognitive Studies, Vol. 2, Deficits in Cognition, pp. 324-337. Brunner/Mazel, New York.

Sapir, S. G., and Nitzburg, A. C. (eds.). 1973. Children with Learning Problems. Brunner/Mazel, New York.

Sapir, S. G., and Wilson, B. 1967. A developmental scale to assist in the prevention of learning disability. In S. G. Sapir and A. C. Nitzburg (eds.), 1973, Children with Learning Problems, pp. 606-612. Brunner/Mazel, New York.

Sapir, S., and Wilson, B. 1978. A Professional's Guide to Working with the Learning-Disabled Child. Brunner/Mazel, New York.

Sass-Kortsak, A. 1975. Wilson's disease: A treatable liver disease in children. Pediatr. Clin. North Am. 22:963-984.

Satterfield, J. H. 1973. EEG issues in children with minimal brain dysfunction. In S. Walzer and P. H. Wolff (eds.), Minimal Cerebral Dysfunction in Children, pp. 35-46. Grune & Stratton, New York.

Satterfield, J. H., Atoian, G., Brashears, G. C., Burleigh, A. C., and Dawson, M. E. 1974. Electrodermal studies in minimal brain dysfunction children. In C. K. Conners (ed.), Clinical Use of Stimulant Drugs in Children, pp. 87-97. Excerpta Medica, Amsterdam.

Satterfield, J. H., Cantwell, D. P., Lesser, L. I., and Podosin, R. L. 1972. Physiological studies of the hyperkinetic child. I. Am. J. Psychiatry 128:1418-1424.

Satterfield, J. H., Cantwell, D. P., and Satterfield, B. T. 1974. Pathophysiology of the hyperactive child syndrome. Arch. Gen. Psychiatry 31:839-844.

Satterfield, J. H., Cantwell, D. P., Saul, R. E., Lesser, L. I., and Podosin, R. L. 1973. Response to stimulant drug treatment in hyperactive children: Prediction from EEG and neurological findings. J. Autism Child Schizophr. 3:36-48.

Satterfield, J., Cantwell, D., Saul, R., and Yusin, A. 1974. Intelligence, academic achievement and EEG abnormalities in hyperactive children. Am. J. Psychiatry 131:391-395.

Satterfield, J. H., Lesser, L. I., Saul, R. E., and Cantwell, D. P. 1973. EEG aspects in the diagnosis and treatment of minimal brain dysfunction. Ann. N.Y. Acad. Sci. 205:274-282.

Sattler, J. M. 1974. Assessment of Children's Intelligence. W. B. Saunders Co., Philadelphia.

Satz, P., and Fletcher, J. M. 1979. Early screening tests: Some uses and abuses. J. Learn. Disabil. 12:56–60.

Satz, P., and Friel, J. 1973. Some predictive antecedents of specific learning disability: A preliminary one-year follow-up. In P. Satz and J. J. Ross (eds.), The Disabled Reader: Early Detection and Intervention, pp. 79–98. Rotterdam University Press, Rotterdam.

Satz, P., and Friel, J. 1978. Predictive validity of an abbreviated screening battery. J. Learn. Disabil. 11:347–351.

Satz, P., and van Nostrand, G. K. 1973. Developmental dyslexia: An evaluation of theory. In P. Satz and J. J. Ross (eds.), The Disabled Reader: Early Detection and Intervention, pp. 121–148. Rotterdam University Press, Rotterdam.

Sauerhoff, M. W., and Michaelson, I. A. 1973. Hyperactivity and brain catecholamines in lead-exposed developing rats. Science 182:1022–1024.

Savage, R. D. 1968. Psychometric Assessment of the Individual Child. Penguin Books, Baltimore.

Savage, R. D., and O'Connor, D. 1966. The assessment of reading and arithmetic retardation in school. Br. J. Educ. Psychol. 34: 317–318.

Schain, R. J. 1972. Neurology of Childhood Learning Disorders. Williams & Wilkins Co., Baltimore.

Schain, R. J. 1973. The neurological evaluation of children with learning disorders. Calif. Med. 118:24–32.

Schain, R. J. 1975. Minimal brain dysfunction. Curr. Probl. Pediatr. 5(10).

Schain, R. J., and Reynard, C. L. 1975. Observations on effects of a central stimulant drug (methylphenidate) in children with hyperactive behavior. Pediatrics 55:709–716.

Schiefelbusch, R. L., and Lloyd, L. L. (eds.). 1974. Language Perspectives—Acquisition, Retardation, and Intervention. University Park Press, Baltimore.

Schiffman, G. 1962. Dyslexia as an educational phenomenon: Its recognition and treatment. In J. Money (ed.), Reading Disability: Progress and Research Needs in Dyslexia, pp. 45–60. Johns Hopkins Press, Baltimore.

Schildkrout, M. S., Shenker, I. R., and Sonnenblick, M. 1972. Human Figure Drawings in Adolescence. Brunner/Mazel, New York.

Schiottz-Christensen, E., and Bruhn, P. 1973. Intelligence, behaviour and scholastic achievement subsequent to febrile convulsions: An analysis of discordant twin-pairs. Dev. Med. Child Neurol. 15:565–575.

Schlager, G., Newman, D. E., Dunn, H. G., Crichton, J. U., and Schulzer, M. 1979. Bone age in children with minimal brain dysfunction. Dev. Med. Child Neurol. 21:41–51.

Schliefer, M., Weiss, G., Cohen, N., Elman, M., Cvejic, H., and Kruger, E. 1975. Hyperactivity in preschoolers and the effect of methylphenidate. Am. J. Orthopsychiatry 45:38–50.

Schmitt, B. 1977. Guidelines for living with a hyperactive child. Pediatrics 60:387.

Schmitt, B. D., Martin, H. P., Nellhaus, T., Cavens, J., Camp, B. W., and Jordan, K. 1973. The hyperactive child. Clin. Pediatr. 12:154–169.

Schnackenberg, R. C. 1973. Caffeine as substitute for Schedule II stimulants in hyperkinetic children. Am. J. Psychiatry 130: 796–798.

Schrag, P. 1975. Readin', Writin' (and Druggin'). New York Times, October 19, p. E13.

Schrag, P., and Divoky, D. 1975. The Myth of the Hyperactive Child. Pantheon Books, New York.

Schroeder, C. S., Schroeder, S. R., and Davine, M. A. 1978. Learning disabilities: Assessment and management of reading problems. In B. B. Wolman (ed.), Handbook of Treatment of Mental Disorders in Childhood and Adolescence, pp. 212–237. Prentice-Hall, Englewood Cliffs, N.J.

Sechzer, J. A., Faro, M. D., and Windle, W. F. 1973. Studies of monkeys asphyxiated at birth: Implications for minimal cerebral dysfunction. In S. Walzer and P. H. Wolff (eds.), Minimal Cerebral Dysfunction in Children, pp. 19–34. Grune & Stratton, New York.

Sells, C. J., Carpenter, R. L., and Ray, C. G. 1975. Sequelae of central-nervous-system enterovirus infections. N. Engl. J. Med. 293:1–4.

Senf, G. M. 1973. Learning disabilities. Pediatr. Clin. North Am. 20:607–640.

Shaywitz, B. A., Cohen, D. J., and Bowers, M. B. 1977. CSF monoamine metabolites in children with minimal brain dysfunction: Evidence for alteration of brain dopamine. J. Pediatr. 90:67–71.

Shaywitz, B. A., Klopper, J. H., and Gordon, J. W. 1978. Methylphenidate in 6-hydroxydopamine treated developing rat pups. Arch. Neurol. 35:463–469.

Shaywitz, B. A., Klopper, J. H., Yager, R. D., and Gordon, J. W. 1976. A paradoxical response to amphetamine in developing rats treated with 6-hydroxydopamine. Nature 261:153–155.

Shaywitz, B. A., Yager, R. D., and Klopper, J. H. 1976. An experimental model of minimal brain dysfunction (MBD) in developing rats. Science 191:305–308.

Shaywitz, S. E., Cohen, D. J., and Shaywitz, B. A. 1978. The biochemical basis of minimal brain dysfunction. J. Pediatr. 92: 179–187.

Shearer, R. B. 1966. Eye findings in children with reading difficulties. J. Pediatr. Ophthalmol. 3:47–53.

Shekim, W. O., Dekirmenjian, H., Chapel, J. L., Javaid, J., and Davis, J. M. 1979. Norepinephrine metabolism and clinical response to dextroamphetamine in hyperactive boys. J. Pediatr. 95:389–394.

Shetty, T. 1971. Alpha rhythms in the hyperkinetic child. Nature 234:476.

Shetty, T. 1973. Some neurologic, electrophysiologic, and biochemical correlates of the hyperkinetic syndrome. Pediatr. Ann. 2(5):29–40.

Shetty, T., and Chase, T. N. 1976. Central monoamines and hyperkinesis of childhood. Neurology 26:1000–1002.

Shields, D. T. 1973. Brain responses to stimuli in disorders of information processing. J. Learn. Disabil. 6:501–505.

Shoumaker, R. D., Bennett, D. R., Bray, P. F., and Curless, R. G. 1974. Clinical and EEG manifestations of an unusual aphasic syndrome in children. Neurology 24:10–16.

Shurin, P. A., Pelton, S. I., Donner, A., and Klein, J. O. 1979. Persistence of middle-ear effusion after acute otitis media in children. N. Engl. J. Med. 300:1121–1123.

Siedentop, K. H., Corrigan, R. A., Loewy, A., and Osenar, S. B. 1978. Eustachian tube function assessed with tympanometry. Ann. Otol. 87:163–169.

Silberberg, N. E., Iversen, I. A., and Goins, J. T. 1973. Which remedial reading method works best? J. Learn. Disabil. 6:547–556.

Silberberg, N., Iversen, I., and Silberberg, M. 1969. A model for classifying children according to their reading level. J. Learn. Disabil. 2:634–643.

Silberberg, N. E., and Silberberg, M. C. 1967. Hyperplexia: Special word recognition skills in young children. Except. Child. 34: 41–42.

Silbergeld, E. K., and Goldberg, A. M. 1974. Lead-induced behavioral dysfunction: An animal model of hyperactivity. Exp. Neurol. 42:146–157.

Silver, A. A. 1950. Diagnostic value of three drawing tests for children. J. Pediatr. 37:129–143.

Silver, A. A. 1961. Diagnostic considerations in children with reading disability. Bull. Orton Soc. 11:5–11.

Silver, A. A., and Hagin, R. A. 1964. Specific reading disability: Follow-up studies. Am. J. Orthopsychiatry 34:95–102.

Silver, A. A., and Hagin, R. A. 1967. Specific reading disability: An approach to diagnosis and treatment. J. Spec. Educ. 1:109–118.

Silver, A. A., Hagin, R. A., DeVito, E., Kreeger, H., and Scully, E. 1976. A search battery for scanning kindergarten children for potential learning disability. J. Am. Acad. Child Psychiatry 15:224–239.

Silver, A. A., Hagin, R. A., and Hersh, M. F. 1967. Reading disability: Teaching through stimulation of deficit perceptual areas. Am. J. Orthopsychiatry 37:744–752.

Silver, L. B. 1971a. Familial patterns in children with neurologically-based learning disabilities. J. Learn. Disabil. 4:349–358.

Silver, L. B. 1971b. The neurologic learning disability syndrome. Am. Fam. Physician 4:95–102.

Silver, L. B. 1971c. A proposed view on the etiology of the neurological learning disability syndrome. J. Learn. Disabil. 4:123–133.

Silver, L. B. 1975. Acceptable and controversial approaches to treating the child with learning disabilities. Pediatrics 55:406–415.

Silverman, L. J., and Metz, A. S. 1973. Numbers of pupils with specific learning disabilities in local public schools in the United States: Spring 1970. Ann N. Y. Acad. Sci. 205:146–157.

Simon, N., and Volicer, L. 1976. Neonatal asphyxia in the rat: Greater vulnerability of males and persistent effects on brain monoamine synthesis. J. Neurochem. 26:893–900.

Skidelsky, R. 1970. English Progressive Schools. Penguin Books, Baltimore.

Sklar, B., Hanley, J., and Simmons, W. W. 1972. An EEG experiment aimed toward identifying dyslexic children. Nature 240:414–416.

Sleator, E. K., and von Neumann, A. W. 1974. Methylphenidate in the treatment of hyperactive children. Clin. Pediatr. 13:19–24.

Sleator, E. K., von Neumann, A., and Sprague, R. L. 1974. Hyperactive children: A continuous long-term placebo-controlled follow-up JAMA 229:316–317.

Smith, C. M. 1971. The relationship of reading method and reading achievement to ITPA sensory modalities. J. Spec. Educ. 5:143–149.

Smith, M. D., Coleman, J. M., Dokecki, R. P., and Davis, E. E. 1977. Recategorized WISC-R scores of learning disabled children. J. Learn. Disabil. 10:437–443.

Smith, F., and Miller, G. A. 1966. The Genesis of Language: A Psycholinguistic Approach. MIT Press, Cambridge, Mass.

Smith, L. H. 1977. Improving Your Child's Behavior Chemistry. Pocket Books, New York.

Smith, P. A., and Marx, R. W. 1972. Some cautions on the use of the Frostig test: A factor analytic study. J. Learn. Disabil. 5:357–362.

Smith, S. L. 1978. No easy Answers: The Learning Disabled Child. HEW/NIMH. DHEW Publication No. (ADM) 77–526.

Snyder, R. D. 1979. The right not to read. Pediatrics 63:791–794.

Snyder, R. D., and Mortimer, J. 1969. Diagnosis and treatment: Dyslexia. Pediatrics 44:601–605.

Snyder, R., and Pope, P. 1970. New norms for and an item analysis of the Wepman test at first-grade, six-year level. Percept. Mot. Skills 31:1007–1010.

Snyder, S. H., and Meyerhoff, J. L. 1973. How amphetamine acts in minimal brain dysfunction. Ann. N.Y. Acad. Sci. 205:310–320.

Sohmer, H., and Student, M. 1978. Auditory nerve and brain-stem evoked response in normal, autistic, minimal brain dysfunction and psychomotor retarded children. Electroencephalogr. Clin. Neurophysiol. 44:380–388.

Solomons, G. 1973. Drug therapy: Initiation and follow-up. Ann. N.Y. Acad. Sci. 205:335–344.

Sorenson, C. A., Vayer, J. S., and Goldberg, C. S. 1977. Amphetamine reduction of motor activity in rats after neonatal administration of 6-hydroxy-dopamine. Biol. Psychiatry 12:133–137.

Sprague, R. L., Barnes, K. R., and Werry, J. S. 1970. Methylphenidate and thioridazine: Learning, reaction time, activity, and classroom behavior in emotionally disturbed children. Am. J. Orthopsychiatry 40:615–628.

Sprague, R. L., and Gadow, K. D. 1976. The role of the teacher in drug treatment. School Rev. 85:109–140.

Sprague, R. L., and Sleator, E. K. 1973. Effects of psychopharmacologic agents on learning disorders. Pediatr. Clin. North Am. 20:719-735.

Sprague, R. L., and Sleator, E. K. 1977. Methylphenidate in hyperkinetic children: Differences in dose effects on learning and social behavior. Science 198:1274-1276.

Sprague, R. L., and Werry, J. S. 1971. Methodology of psychopharmacological studies with the retarded. In N. R. Ellis (ed.), International Review of Research in Mental Retardation, Vol. 5, pp. 148-219. Academic Press, New York.

Spring, C., and Sandoval, J. 1976. Food additives and hyperkinesis: A critical evaluation of the evidence. J. Learn. Disabil. 9: 560-569.

Stainback, S. B., Stainback, W. C., and Hallahan, D. P. 1973. Effect of background music on learning. Except. Child. 40:109-110.

Steg, J. P., and Rapoport, J. L. 1975. Minor physical anomalies in normal, neurotic, learning disabled, and severely disturbed children. J. Autism Child. Schizophr. 5:299-307.

Steinberg, D. D., and Yamada, J. 1978. Are whole word Kanji easier to learn than syllable Kana? Read. Res. Quart. 14:88-99.

Steinberg, M., and Rendle-Short, J. 1977. Vestibular dysfunction in young children with minor neurological impairment. Dev. Med. Child Neurol. 19:639-651.

Stevens, J. R., Sachdev, K., and Milstein, V. 1968. Behavior disorders of childhood and the electroencephalogram. Arch. Neurol. 18:160-177.

Stevenson, H. W., Parker, T., Wilkinson, A., Bonnevaux, B., and Gonzalez, M. 1978. Schooling, environment, and cognitive development: A cross-cultural study. Monogr. Soc. Res. Child Dev. 43(3)(serial no. 175).

Stewart, M. A., and Morrison, J. R. 1973. Affective disorder among the relatives of hyperactive children. J. Child Psychol. Psychiatry 14:209-212.

Stewart, M. A., Pitts, F. N., Craig, A. G., and Dieruf, W. 1966. The hyperactive child syndrome. Am. J. Orthopsychiatry 36:861-867.

Sticht, T. G., Caylor, J. S., Kern, R. P., and Fox, L. C. 1972. Project REALISTIC: Determination of adult functional literacy skill levels. Read. Res. Quart. 7:424-465.

Stockard, J. J., Stockard, J. E., and Sharbrough, F. W. 1978. Non-pathologic factors influencing brain stem auditory evoked potentials. Am. J. EEG Technol. 18:177-209.

Stores, G. 1978. School-childrer with epilepsy at risk for learning and behaviour problems. Dev. Med. Child Neurol. 20:502-508.

Stores, G., and Hart, J, 1976. Reading skills of children with generalized or focal epilepsy attending ordinary school. Dev. Med. Child Neurol. 18:705-716.

Strauss, A. A., and Lehtinen, L. 1947. Psychopathology and Education of the Brain Injured Child. Grune & Stratton, New York.

Strauss, A. A., and Werner, H. 1942. Disorders of conceptual thinking in the brain-injured child. J. Nerv. Ment. Dis. 96:153-172.

Stroufe, L. A., and Stewart, M. A. 1973. Treating problem children with stimulant drugs. N. Engl. J. Med. 289:407-413.

Surwillo, W. W. 1977. Changes in the electroencephalogram accompanying the use of stimulant drugs (methylphenidate and dextroamphetamine) in hyperactive children. Biol. Psychiatry 12:787-799.

Swanson, J. M., and Kinsbourne, M. 1976. Stimulant-related state-dependent learning in hyperactive children. Science 192:1354-1357.

Swanson, J., Kinsbourne, M., Roberts, W., and Zucker, K. 1978. Time-response analysis of the effect of stimulant medication on the learning ability of children referred for hyperactivity. Pediatrics 61:21-29.

Swanson, W. I. 1972. Optometric vision therapy—How successful is it in the treatment of learning disorders? J. Learn. Disabil. 5:285-290.

Szasz, T. 1974. Ceremonial Chemistry. Anchor Press, Garden City, N.Y.

Talbot, M. E. 1964. Edouard Sequin: A Study of An Educational Approach to the Treatment of Mentally Defective Children. Teachers College Press, New York.

Tarnopol, L. (ed.). 1969a. Learning Disabilities. Charles C Thomas Publisher, Springfield, Ill.

Tarnopol, L. 1969b. Introduction to children with learning disabilities. In L. Tarnopol (ed.), Learning Disabilities, pp. 5-30. Charles C Thomas Publisher, Springfield, Ill.

Tarnopol, L. 1969c. Delinquency and learning disabilities. In L. Tarnopol (ed.), Learning Disabilities, pp. 305-330. Charles C Thomas Publishers, Springfield, Ill.

Tarver, S. G., and Dawson, M. M. 1978. Modality preference and the teaching of reading: A review. J. Learn. Disabil. 11:5-17.

Taylor, E. M. 1961. Psychological Appraisal of Children with Cerebral Defects. Harvard University Press, Cambridge, Mass.

Templin, M. C. 1966. The study of articulation and language development during the early school years. In S. Smith and G. A. Miller (eds.), The Genesis of Language, pp. 173-180. MIT Press, Cambridge, Mass.

Thomas, A., and Chess, S. 1977. Temperament and Development. Brunner/Mazel, New York.

Tiwary, C. M., Rosenbloom, A. L., Robertson, M .F., and Parker, J. C. 1975. Effects of thyrotropin-releasing hormone in minimal brain dysfunction. Pediatrics 56:119-121.

Touwen, B. C. L. 1972. Laterality and dominance. Dev. Med. Child. Neurol. 14:747-755.

Touwen, B. C. L. 1979. Examination of the Child with Minor Neurological Dysfunction. Clinics in Developmental Medicine No. 71. J. B. Lippincott Co., Philadelphia.

Touwen, B. C. L., and Prechtl, H. F. R. 1970. The Neurological Examination of the Child with Minor Nervous Dysfunction. Clinics in Developmental Medicine No. 38. Spastics Society Medical Education and Information Unit in association with William Heinemann Medical Books, Ltd., London.

Touwen, B. C. L., and Sporrel, T. 1979. Soft signs and MBD. Dev. Med. Child Neurol. 21:528-530.

Towbin, A. 1971. Organic causes of minimal brain dysfunction: Perinatal origin of minimal cerebral lesions. JAMA 217:1207-1214.

Twitchell, T. E., Lecours, A.-R., Rudel, R. G., and Teuber, H.-L. 1966. Minimal cerebral dysfunction in children: Motor deficits. Trans. Am. Neurol. Assoc. 91:353-355.

Ungerstedt, U. 1971. Stereotaxic mapping of the monamine pathways in the rat brain. Acta Physiol. Scand. 367 (suppl.): 1-48.

Vance, H., Wallbrown, F. H., and Blaha, J. 1978. Determining WISC-R profiles for reading disabled children. J. Learn. Disabil. 11:657-661.

Van Osdon, B. M., Johnson, D. M., and Geiger, L. 1974. The effects of total body movement on reading achievement. Aust. J. Ment. Retard. 3:16-19.

Varga, J. 1979. The hyperactive child: Should we be paying more attention? Am. J. Dis. Child. 133:413–418.

Vaughan, R., and Hodges, L. 1973. A statistical survey into a definition: A search for acceptance. J. Learn. Disabil. 6:658–664.

Vellutino, F. R. 1977. Alternative conceptualizations of dyslexia: Evidence in support of a verbal-deficit hypothesis. Harvard Educ. Rev. 47:334–354.

Vellutino, F. R., Bentley, W. L., and Phillips, F. 1978. Inter-versus intrahemispheric learning in dyslexic and normal readers. Dev. Med. Child Neurol. 20:71–80.

Vellutino, F., Smith, H., Steger, J., and Kaman, M. 1975. Reading disabilities: Age differences and the perceptual-deficit hypothesis. Child Dev. 46:487–493.

Vellutino, F., Steger, J., and Kandel, G. 1972. Reading disability: An investigation of the perceptual deficit hypothesis. Cortex 8:106–118.

Vellutino, F. R., Steger, B. M., Moyer, S. C., Harding, C. J., and Niles, J. A. 1977. Has the perceptual deficit hypothesis led us astray? J. Learn. Disabil. 10:375–385.

Vernon, M. D. 1977. Varieties of deficiency in the reading process. Harvard Educ. Rev. 47:396–410.

Vogel, S. A. 1975. Syntactic Abilities in Normal and Dyslexic Children. University Park Press, Baltimore.

Vuckovich, D. M. 1968. Pediatric neurology and learning disabilities. In H. R. Myklebust (ed.), Progress in Learning Disabilities, Vol. 1, pp. 16–38. Grune & Stratton, New York.

Vygotsky, L. S. 1962. Thought and Language. MIT Press, Cambridge, Mass.

Waber, D. P. 1979. Neuropsychological aspects of Turner's syndrome. Dev. Med. Child Neurol. 21:58–70.

Wade, M. G. 1976. Effects of methylphenidate on motor skill acquisition of hyperactive children. J. Learn. Disabil. 9:443–447.

Wagenheim, L. 1959. Learning problems associated with childhood diseases contracted at age two. Am. J. Orthopsychiatry 29:102–109.

Waldrop, M. F., Bell, R. Q., McLaughlin, B., and Halverson, C. F., Jr. 1978. Newborn minor physical anomalies predict short attention span, peer aggression, and impulsivity at age 3. Science 199:563–565.

Waldrop, M. F., and Goering, J. D. 1971. Hyperactivity and minor physical anomalies in elementary school children. Am. J. Orthopsychiatry 41:602-607.

Waldrop, M. F., and Halverson, C. F., Jr. 1971. Minor physical anomalies and hyperactive behavior in young children. In J. Hellmuth (ed.), Exceptional Infant, Vol. 2, Studies in Abnormalities, pp. 343-380. Brunner/Mazel, New York.

Waldrop, M., Pedersen, F., and Bell, R. 1968. Minor physical anomalies and behavior in preschool children. Child Dev. 39:391-400.

Walker, W., Ellis, M. I., Ellis, E., Curry, A., Savage, R. D., and Sawyer, R. 1974. A follow-up study of survivors of Rh-haemolytic disease. Dev. Med. Child Neurol. 16:592-611.

Wallace, S. J., and Cull, A. M. 1979. Long-term psychological outlook for children whose first fit occurs with fever. Dev. Med. Child Neurol. 21:28-40.

Walzer, S., and Richmond, J. B. 1973. The epidemiology of learning disorders. Pediatr. Clin. North Am. 20:549-565.

Walzer, S., and Wolff, P. H. (eds.). 1973. Minimal Cerebral Dysfunction in Children. Grune & Stratton, New York.

Ward, W. D., and Barcher, P. R. 1975. Reading achievement and creativity as related to open classroom experience. J. Educ. Psychol. 67:683-691.

Warren, R. J., Karduck, W. A., Bussaratid, S., Stewart, M. A., and Sly, W. S. 1971. The hyperactive child syndrome: Normal chromosome findings. Arch. Gen. Psychiatry 24:161-162.

Waugh, R. P. 1973. The relationship between individual modality preference and performance after four instructional procedures. Except. Child. 39:465-469.

Wechsler, D. 1974. Manual for the Wechsler Intelligence Scale for Children—Revised. Psychological Corporation, New York.

Wedell, K. 1960. Variations in perceptual ability among types of cerebral palsy. Cerebr. Palsy Bull. 2:149-157.

Weil, A. P. 1970. Children with minimal brain dysfunction: Diagnostic, dynamic and therapeutic considerations. In S. G. Sapir and A. C. Nitzburg (eds.), 1973. Children with Learning Problems, pp. 551-568. Brunner/Mazel, New York.

Weiss, G., Kruger, E., Danielson, U., and Elman, M. 1975. Effect of long-term treatment of hyperactive children with methylphenidate. Can. Med. Assoc. J. 112:159-165.

Weiss, G., Minde, K., Werry, J. S., Douglas, V., and Nemeth, E. 1971. Studies on the hyperactive child: Five-year follow-up. Arch. Gen. Psychiatry 24:409–414.

Welner, Z., Welner, A., Stewart, M., Palkes, H., and Wish, E. 1977. A controlled study of siblings of hyperactive children. J. Nerv. Ment. Dis. 165:110–117.

Wender, E. H. 1977. Food additives and hyperkinesis. Am. J. Dis. Child. 131:1204–1206.

Wender, P. H. 1971. Minimal Cerebral Dysfunction in Children. Wiley-Interscience, New York.

Wender, P. 1972. The minimal brain dysfunction syndrome in children. J. Nerv. Ment. Dis. 155:55–71.

Wender, P. 1973a. Minimal brain dysfunction: Some recent advances. Pediatr. Ann. 2(5):42–54.

Wender, P. H. 1973b. Some speculations concerning a possible biochemical basis of minimal brain dysfunction. Ann. N.Y. Acad. Sci. 205:18–28.

Wepman, J. M. 1958. Auditory Discrimination Test. Language Research Associates, Chicago.

Wepman, J. M. 1962. Dyslexia: Its relationship to language acquisition and concept formation. In J. Money (ed.), Reading Disability: Progress and Research Needs in Dyslexia, pp. 179–186. Johns Hopkins Press, Baltimore.

Werner, E. E., and Smith, R. S. 1977. Kauai's Children Come of Age. University of Hawaii Press, Honolulu.

Werry, J. S. 1968a. Developmental hyperactivity. Pediatr. Clin. North Am. 15:581–599.

Werry, J. S. 1968b. Studies on the hyperactive child. IV. An empirical analysis of the minimal brain dysfunction syndrome. Arch. Gen. Psychiatry 19:9–16.

Werry, J. S., Aman, M. G., and Lampen, E. 1976. Haloperidol and methylphenidate in hyperactive children. Acta Paedopsychiatrica 42:26–40.

Werry, J. S., Minde, K., Guzman, A., Weiss, G., Dogan, K., and Hoy, E. 1972. Studies on the hyperactive child. VII. Neurological status compared with neurotic and normal children. Am. J. Orthopsychiatry 42:441–450.

Werry, J. S., Weiss, G., Douglas, V., and Martin, J. 1966. Studies on the hyperactive child. III. The effects of chlorpromazine upon behaviour and learning ability. J. Am. Acad. Child Psychiatry 5:292–312.

Werry, J. S., and Wollersheim, J. P. 1967. Behavior therapy with children: A broad overview. J. Am. Acad. Child Psychiatry 7: 346–370.

Whalen, C. K., and Henker, B. 1976. Psychostimulants and children: A review and analysis. Psychol. Bull. 83:1113–1130.

Wheatley, M. D. 1944. The hypothalamus and affective behavior in cats. A study of the effects of experimental lesions, with anatomic correlations. Arch. Neurol. Psychiatry 52:296–316.

White, J. H. 1977. Pediatric Psychopharmacology. Williams & Wilkins Co., Baltimore.

Whiton, M. B., Singer, D. L., and Cook, H. 1975. Sensory integration skills as predictors of reading acquisition. J. Read. Behav. 7:79–90.

Wiener, G., Rider, R. V., Oppel, W. C., Fischer, L. K., and Harper, P. A. 1965. Correlates of low birth weight: Psychological status at six to seven years of age. Pediatrics 35:434–444.

Wiener, J. M. (ed.). 1977. Psychopharamcology in Childhood and Adolescence. Basic Books, New York.

Wigglesworth, R. 1961. Minimal cerebral palsy. Cerebr. Palsy Bull. 3:293–295.

Wigglesworth, R. 1963. The importance of recognizing minimal cerebral dysfunction in pediatric practice. In R. MacKeith and M. Bax (eds.), Minimal Cerebral Dysfunction, pp. 34–38. Spastics Society Medical Education and Information Unit in association with William Heinemann Medical Books, Ltd., London.

Wikler, A., Dixon, J. F., and Parker, J. B., Jr. 1970. Brain function in problem children and controls: Psychometric, neurological, and electroencephalographic comparisons. Am. J. Psychiatry 127:634–645.

Willerman, L. 1973. Activity level and hyperactivity in twins. Child Dev. 44:288–293.

Williams, J. I., Cram, D. M., Tausig, F. T., and Webster, E. 1978. Relative effects of drugs and diet on hyperactive behaviors: An experimental study. Pediatrics 61:811–817.

Windle, W. F. 1968. Brain damage at birth. JAMA 206:1967–1972.

Winet, R. A., and Wikler, R. C. 1972. Current behavior modification in the classroom: Be still, be quiet, be docile. J. Appl. Behav. Anal. 5:499–504.

Winsberg, B. G., Press, M., Bialer, I., and Kupietz, S. 1974. Dextroamphetamine and methylphenidate in the treatment of hyperactive/aggressive children. Pediatrics 53:236–241.

Witelson, S. 1976. Sex and the single hemisphere: Specialization of the right hemisphere for spatial processing. Science 193:425–427.

Witelson, S. 1977. Developmental dyslexia: Two right hemispheres and none left. Science 195:309–311.

Witelson, S. F., and Rabinovitch, M. S. 1972. Hemispheric speech lateralization in children with auditory-linguistic defects. Cortex 8:412–426.

Witkin, H. A., Mednick, S. A., Schulsinger, F., Bakkestrom, E., Christiansen, K. O., Goodenough, D. R., Hirschhorn, K., Lundsteen, C., Owen, D. R., Philip, J., Rubin, D. B., and Stocking, M. 1976. Criminality in XYY and XXY men. Science 193:547–555.

Wolcott, G. J. 1972. Learning disability: A cooperative team approach. Wis. Med. J. 71:223–226.

Wolf, T. 1977. Reading reconsidered. Harvard Educ. Rev. 47: 411–429.

Wolff, P. H. 1969. What we must and must not teach our young children from what we know about early cognitive development. In P. Wolff and R. MacKeith (eds.), Planning for Better Learning, pp. 7–19. Spastics Society Medical Education and Information Unit in association with William Heinemann Medical Books, Ltd., London.

Wolff, P. H., and Hurwitz, I. 1966. The choreiform syndrome. Dev. Med. Child Neurol. 8:160–165.

Wolff, P. H., and Hurwitz, I. 1973. Functional implications of the minimal brain damage syndrome. In S. Walzer and P. H. Wolff (eds.), Minimal Cerebral Dysfunction in Children, pp. 105–115. Grune & Stratton, New York.

Wolff, P. H., and MacKeith, R. (eds.). 1969. Planning for Better Learning. Clinics in Developmental Medicine No. 33. Spastics Society Medical Education and Information Unit in association with William Heinemann Medical Books, Ltd., London.

Wolff, P., and Wolff, E. A. 1972. Correlational analysis of motor and verbal activity in young children. Child Dev. 43:1407–1411.

Wolraich, M. L. 1977. Stimulant drug therapy in hyperactive children: Research and clinical implications. Pediatrics 60:512–518.

Wright, B. J., and Isenstein, V. R. 1977. Psychological Tests and Minorities. Mental Health Studies and Reports Branch, U.S. Government Printing Office, Washington, D.C.

Yahraes, H., and Prestwich, S. 1976. Detection and Prevention of Learning Disorders. DHEW Publication No. (ADM) 77-337.

Yepes, L. E., Balka, E. B., Winsberg, B. G., and Bialer, I. 1977. Amitriptyline and methylphenidate treatment of behaviorally disordered children. J. Child Psychol. Psychiatry 18:39–52.

Yule, W. 1967. Predicting reading ages on Neale's analysis of reading ability. Br. J. Educ. Psychol. 37:252–255.

Yule, W. 1973. Differential prognosis of reading backwardness and specific reading retardation. Br. J. Educ. Psychol. 43:244–248.

Yule, W. 1976. Issues and problems in remedial education. Dev. Med. Child Neurol. 18:674–682.

Zangwill, O. L. 1962. Dyslexia in relation to cerebral dominance. In J. Money (ed.), Reading Disability: Progress and Research Needs in Dyslexia, pp. 103–113. Johns Hopkins Press, Baltimore.

Zangwill, O. L. 1963. The cerebral localization of psychological function. Adv. Sci. 20:335–344.

Zarin-Ackerman, J., Lewis, M., and Driscoll, J. M. 1977. Language development in 2-year-old normal and risk infants. Pediatrics 59:982–986.

Zigler, E., and Seitz, V. 1975. On "An experimental evaluation of sensorimotor patterning": A critique. Am. J. Ment. Defic. 79:483–492.

Zinkus, P. W., Gottlieb, M. I., Schapiro, M. 1978. Developmental and psychoeducational sequelae of chronic otitis media. Am. J. Dis. Child. 132:1100–1104.

INDEX

Syndrome—*cont.*
 choreiform, 3, 84, 97, 98
 clumsy child, 3, 7, 95, 105
 fetal alcohol, 55
 47XYY, 53
 frontal lobe, 42, 120
 Gerstmann, 6, 34, 52
 Gilles de la Tourette, 146
 Klinefelter, 53
 Klippel-Feil, 95
 Strauss, 19
 Turner, 53
Synkinesia, 95, 96, 99, 101

Teacher, 24, 51, 88–89, 175, 176, 184
Teeth, 104
Temporal lobe, 41, 146
Tension fatigue syndrome, 57
Testes, undescended, 104
Tests
 Bender-Gestalt, 33, 53, 120, 147
 Draw A Person (DAP), 119, 120
 Face-Hand, 102
 Finger to Nose, 102
 Fog, 99–101
 Photo-Metrazol Activation, 113
 Schilder's, 97
 Visual Aural Digit Span (VADS), 121–126
Thalidomide, 70
Thioridazine (Mellaril), 140
Tonic labyrinthine reflex, 104
TORCH, 64
Treatment
 educational, 172–174
 perceptual motor, 69–78
 see also Behavioral psychology; Drugs; Stimulants

Turner syndrome, 53
Tutoring, 129
Twin studies, 52

Underachievement, *see* School failure
Underarousal, 42, 112, 113, 135
 see also Attention; Diencephalon
Undescended testes, 104

Verbal-Performance (V-P) discrepancies, 7, 12, 70, 160–163
Vestibular dysfunction, 63, 104
Visual aural digit span (VADS), 121–126
Visual deficit, 3, 29, 30, 59–61
Visual evoked response (VER), 113, 114
Visual perception, 73, 74

Wechsler Intelligence Scale for Children-Revised (WISC-R), 52, 57, 155–167
 subscore scatter, 4, 7, 163–166
 verbal-performance (V-P) discrepancies, 7, 12, 70, 160–163
Wepman, 74
Writing problems, *see* Dysgraphia

Z-score discrepancy method, 197, 198